THE CHEMISTRY OF CONSCIOUS STATES

Also by J. Allan Hobson

The Dreaming Brain
Sleep

The Chemistry of
Conscious States

How the Brain Changes Its Mind

J. Allan Hobson, M.D.

Little, Brown and Company

BOSTON   NEW YORK   TORONTO   LONDON

First Edition

Library of Congress Cataloging-in-Publication Data

Hobson, J. Allan.
    The chemistry of conscious states: how the brain changes its mind / by J. Allan Hobson. — 1st ed.
            p.   cm.
Includes index.
ISBN 0-316-36754-0
1. Consciousness — Physiological aspects.   2. Neuropsychology.
    3. Neurochemistry.   I. Title.
    QP411.H63   1994
    612.8'2 — dc20   94-15538

10   9   8   7   6   5   4   3   2   1

HAD
Published simultaneously in Canada by
Little, Brown & Company (Canada) Limited

Printed in the United States of America

*To all those patients, students, and colleagues
who have so greatly enriched my scientific life
by becoming my collaborators in brain-mind
research*

The Brain — is wider than the Sky —
    For — put them side by side —
The one the other will contain
    With ease — and You — beside —

The Brain is deeper than the sea —
    For — hold them — Blue to Blue —
The one the other will absorb —
    As Sponges — Buckets — do —

The Brain is just the weight of God —
    For — Heft them — Pound for Pound —
And they will differ — if they do —
    As Syllable from Sound —

                        Emily Dickinson

CONTENTS

ACKNOWLEDGMENTS

The Chemistry of Conscious States builds upon the science out-lined in *The Dreaming Brain* and *Sleep* but is different from those books in three major respects. The first is its emphasis upon our recent and systematic research on dreaming. The second is its use of experiential details from my own life and the lives of my pa-tients. And the third is its greatly enlarged scope that now includes speculations about consciousness itself.

Except for coworkers and colleagues of the author, pseudonyms have been used to protect the privacy of certain individuals, and, in some cases, composites have been drawn from several individu-als for brevity and clarity.

The new research on dreaming was carried out by a team of co-workers most of whom were students in the course Waking, Sleep-ing and Dreaming that I have taught in the Harvard Extension School since 1989. This team, which has met as the Wednesday Dream Seminar for the past five years, includes David Kahn, Jane Merritt, Edward Pace-Schott, Jeff Sutton, Richie Davidson, Jody Resnick, Cindy Rittenhouse, and Bob Stickgold. Our most glori-ous joint achievement has been the publication of eight articles on dreaming that filled an entire issue of the journal *Consciousness and Cognition* earlier this year.

For over thirty years I have been privileged to work at the Massachusetts Mental Health Center, where the personal experiences of patients were our most highly valued data. From the time of my residency training in psychiatry through my quarter century as clinician and scientist, I have been able to elicit and attend to descriptions of conscious states in all their glorious variety and detail from a veritable legion of informants. I cannot name the individual patients who helped me get the sense of the neuropathology of everyday life that I try to convey in this book. Many of them will recognize their contributions, and I hope all of them will accept my respectful thanks.

The courage to tackle the dauntingly broad and deep subject of consciousness grew out of my participation in the Mind-Body Network of the John D. and Catherine T. MacArthur Foundation. This network (which was the brainchild of Jonas Salk, Murray Gill-Mann, Peter Nathan, and Denis Prager) has been one of the most stimulating intellectual experiences of my life. From such bright and creative thinkers as Ken Hugdahl, David Spiegel, Ann Harrington, Eve VanCauter, Phil Gold, Mardi Horowitz, Steven Kosslyn, and Bob Rose, I have learned many of the facts and concepts that are the fabric of the middle of the book. The resources of the foundation have also materially aided my research by complementing my support from the NIMH in an encouraging way.

Conscious States has been in the making since 1991. Jill Kneerim and Ike Williams of the Palmer and Dodge Agency helped me get the project rolling and offered their wise counsel when roadblocks appeared. I wrote the first draft while serving as a visiting professor in the Neurology Department of the University of Messina in Sicily. My hosts Raoul di Perri and Lia Sylvestri helped me in three ways: they made sure my formal academic responsibilities were light; they lent me their beachfront condominium near Taormina; and they offered me their gracious good company on many memorable social occasions. Learning to cook risotto was an unanticipated fringe benefit of my Sicilian sojourn.

Translating my abstruse and jargon-filled prose was the joint effort of Jordan Pavlin and Bill Phillips, my editors at Little, Brown, and of Mark Fischetti, a journalist who knows how to turn the densest science writing into lucid narrative. Any opacity that still clouds this book's messages is my responsibility, not theirs.

In preparing the manuscript, I had the assistance of Jane Merritt, who typed the first draft from my 450-page longhand journal, and Dolly Abbott, who organized the many revisions that have since been necessary.

Now I can only hope that you will be an active and critical reader. Please send me any questions, ideas, or accounts of your own conscious states that this book may inspire.

ALLAN HOBSON
Boston, Massachusetts

PART ONE

DEFINING THE BRAIN-MIND

CHAPTER 1

The Brain Is Insane

I MUCH PREFER old hotels to modern ones, and one look around the charming lobby I was now standing in made me happy. My New Orleans host had heeded my request to be billeted simply during the important scientific meeting I was to attend here. But as I stepped into an adjoining room, I suddenly realized that I had stumbled upon a crime in progress. The easy comfort of my exploratory prowl turned to dread panic. My heart pounded in my chest, and my stomach churned in fear.

My first impulse was to run for it, but since the security guard across the room was aiming his shotgun in my direction, I froze. Then I watched in fearful fascination as he slowly turned his weapon upward toward the ceiling, zeroing in on unseen intruders. I was relieved to realize that at least the guard had not mistaken *me* for one of *them*. Beckoning me not to move and to keep silent, the guard advanced to the center of the room and trained his gaze back on the ceiling above the door I had just entered. What is he noticing? I wondered as my eyes and ears at first detected no evidence of a target.

Then it all became quite clear. The weapon I had mistaken for a shotgun was actually an ingenious electronic detection device that was picking up and amplifying voices emanating from the room above. As the guard swept his invisible electronic beam back and forth along the ceiling, he focused on two clearly audible voices about six feet apart. Each voice was that of a man, speaking as though he had no idea he could be overheard and discussing details of the hotel break-in he and his accomplice had engineered. Although the voices were easily understood, and although the language specifically described the criminals' strategy, I could not make any sense of what was said. It was almost as if the meaning of the sentences, if there was any, dissolved immediately upon their utterance.

No matter that I can't comprehend their dialogue, I thought, the key is to localize the culprits so that they can be apprehended. To accomplish this goal, the guard mounted a stepladder and drew two circles on the ceiling with a large felt-tipped marker. That's exactly where they are, I realized, as if the circles would facilitate the thieves' arrest by police, who I imagined must be closing in on them in the room above.

Within what must have been considerably less than a second, this gripping mystery thriller gave way to quite a different scenario: the gray dawn of a foggy, rainy Monday morning in Ogunquit, Maine, the tail end of a long and restful Fourth of July weekend. I chuckled as I rolled over beneath my blanket because the plot of my little dream had been so beguiling and because, once again, I had been so completely fooled by it.

You need quite a good sense of humor to deal with the reality of dreaming, I thought, because it is clear that you are as crazy as a loon when you are in the grips of a dream. There is no madness more delirious than dreaming, I realized once again for the umpteenth time.

Only seconds before I awakened to the pitter-patter of the raindrops outside my window, I had been completely convinced of the reality of a wild world of impossibly fluid visual imagery (in which a gun became a voice detector), of impossibly keen auditory analysis (in which voices were heard but speech was not recognized), of inconsistent and uncanny logic (in which unseen intruders were remotely localized and encircled), and of paralytic anxiety (in which no matter how scared I was I could not run). I have had even more impossible dreams, but even then I usually haven't caught on to the fact that I was dreaming.

What is the difference between my dreams and madness? What is the difference between my dream experience and the waking experience of someone who is psychotic, demented, or just plain crazy? In terms of the nature of the experience, there is none. In my New Orleans dream I hallucinated: I saw and heard things that weren't in my bedroom. I was deluded: I believed that the dream actions were real despite gross internal inconsistencies. I was disoriented: I believed that I was in an old hotel in New Orleans when I was actually in a house in Ogunquit. I was illogical: I believed that drawing circles on a ceiling would help police localize individuals in a room above. I was emotionally seized: I was so dominated by my sudden fear that my guts were convulsed and my senses driven to insane contrivance. And I was confabulating: I was telling myself a story in order to integrate my hallucinations, my delusions, my emotions, and my deranged analytical powers.

Once I woke up, I was not worried about my temporary insanity. My dream was no more ludicrous than any other dream I have had. And I'll bet you've had some yourself that were much more bizarre. We all take comfort in our conviction that our nightly madness is an important function of that incredible handful of jelly that lies behind our eyes and between our ears. I am talking, of course, about our brains.

I have been thinking about my brain for some time now, and I'm beginning to realize something that seems to me to be quite startling and important. And that is that I can no longer make any meaningful distinction between the state of my brain and the state of my mind. Especially when I consider dreaming.

DREAMING AS DELIRIUM

As I lay in my Ogunquit bed dreaming about the detection of criminals in a hotel in New Orleans, I was so convinced by the reality of my subjective experience that I believed myself to be awake. Thus, I was in no position to deduce anything valid about the state of my consciousness.

Within an instant, however, my brain state changed from dreaming to waking. I immediately knew that it was Monday, July 5, 1992 (not October 10, 1991, the time of the dream) and that I was in Ogunquit, Maine, not New Orleans, Louisiana. Awake, I was oriented, not disoriented. Awake, my plan for the day was logical and clear, not confused and cloudy. And yet the dream state affected my waking state. My memory of the dream, although fragmented, was vivid and detailed after I had awakened, and I can recall it just as clearly now, some twenty-four hours later, as clearly as I can all my subsequent actions of yesterday, when I drove with my son from Ogunquit to my farmhouse here in the hills of northern Vermont. This is odd, because all the other dreams I had had that Sunday night, and the ninety thousand others I have had during the nights' sleep of my life, are utterly lost to a massive and everlasting amnesia.

It seems indubitable that the sharp and dramatic change in my mental state was caused by an equally sharp and dramatic change in my brain state, from sleep to awake. It is this perfect match of brain state to mind state that gives me the courage to propose that it is an error to use two different sets of words, concepts, and feelings when considering our brains (on the one hand) and our minds (on the other). I believe that the brain and the mind are inextricably bound. There is no difference between the physical brain in my skull and the allegedly ethereal mind that floats about me in some fifth dimension none of us can observe. The brain and mind constitute an inseparable unity.

My conviction that the brain and mind are one springs from the recognition that the nature of each state of consciousness that I experience subjectively is determined by the state of my brain. I dream because something specific is happening among the neurons in my brain. I wake up because that activity suddenly changes again in a specific manner. Therefore I propose that we call this unity the brain-mind and that we refer to its major modes of operation — like dreaming and waking — as brain-mind states.

Although this idea may seem logical and harmless enough, it is no less than heresy to both science and the humanities. Many scientists describe the brain as a biological central processor and deny the existence of mind. And many humanists describe the mind as some glorious entity — a being unto itself, a self-aware spirit that transcends any physical embodiment. Thus we are portrayed as mindless brains or brainless minds, and never the twain shall meet. The brain runs the body — it enables us to see, to walk, to digest our food. The mind runs our thoughts and personalities — it enables us to think, to feel, to judge our surroundings and the people in them.

But I have come to believe that the brain and the mind are not two entities linked in some lucky cosmic way. They are one entity. And the normal modes of experience that make up our lives, like waking and dreaming, and those abnormal modes suffered by some of us, like schizophrenia and the DTs, are simply different *states* of the brain-mind, whether healthy or not.

This hypothesis is not something I have pulled from thin air. Trained in both neurology (the "brain camp") and psychiatry (the "mind camp"), I have studied people for more than thirty years with a dual insight. Recent years have brought great advances in both fields, thanks to new diagnostic technology such as magnetic resonance imaging (MRI), the gathering of empirical data on what goes on in our heads when we sleep and dream, and medical discoveries about such diseases as Alzheimer's. The new ideas coming from these advances are all converging to one common understanding: that there is a unified brain-mind.

I call this new way of looking at things the brain-mind paradigm. I use the hyphenated term "brain-mind" to denote unity. And I use the word "paradigm" to denote a new and explicit model of that unity. As Thomas Kuhn has pointed out, a paradigm shift is more than an incremental change in the status of a scientific theory; it is a revolutionary change in our way of seeing and understanding our world and, in this case, it is a revolutionary way of understanding ourselves.

In Part One, I intend to lay this theory out for you in detail. Where does it come from? Why is it so compelling? Why is it so exciting? And so shocking? Why do I say that there is not simply an analogy between, say, dreaming and psychosis, but that dreaming and psychosis are the same kinds of things — similar variants of brain-mind state? To you, a "normal" person, a dream is regular behavior. To a psychotic, an episode of hallucination is just as routine. The new brain-mind theory is not complete, but it is being fine-tuned every day in labs and hospitals where normal and abnormal people go to be studied and cured.

This book is not about the strange experiences of a few people. It is about the strangeness of the experience of all people, so it is a book about you. And while I do not intend to take away any reverent sense you may have about your own dreams, or your spirit, or your soul, I do intend to help you understand all your experiences in terms of brain-mind states.

Part Two introduces the major faculties of the mind — orientation, memory, perception, emotion, attention, and mood — and shows how these are all a function of, and are all dependent on, the state of the brain-mind. It discusses how brain-mind states function, how they change, and what makes them change. Why you may be confused when you wake up from sleep. Why your aging parent with Alzheimer's or your son with attention deficit disorder may suddenly switch from lucid conversation to an aloof stare.

And here's the powerful punchline — the payoff — to you, to me, and to those misunderstood men and women in mental institutions around the world: if we can explain how the brain-mind controls these faculties, then we can improve our own lives and those of others. You will see in Part Three that you can improve your health, your sleep, your memory, and your ability to learn, by voluntarily controlling your brain-mind state. You will also begin to understand the frightful behavior of people with "mental problems" and will see that there are sound ways to help them rectify their own mixed-up brain-mind states. I hope, too, you will come to agree that it is extremely important to bring back together the neurologists and the psychiatrists — the scientists and the humanists — to a shared vision and thus a shared pursuit of better mental and physical well-being for all of us.

So come with me on this brain-mind odyssey.

THE FIRST time I began to think that there might be a way of scientifically establishing brain-mind unity was during my medical internship at Bellevue Hospital in New York City, in 1960. In that year I saw hundreds of cases of so-called mental illness that were actually caused by brain disease.

As anyone who grew up in the New York area knows, the name Bellevue is synonymous with nuthouse, loony bin, and mental hospital. Some people just call it The Psycho. Kids say to each other "Stop being goofy or they'll send you to Bellevue." When I was there, Bellevue was the triage center for every man, woman, and child who acted crazy on the streets of Manhattan south of Forty-second Street and east of Fifth Avenue. That's nutty territory on the best of days.

If a person was wildly psychotic and out of control when he entered the Bellevue Psycho admissions unit, he would be labeled schizophrenic and sent up to the ninth floor of the psychiatry building for confinement and observation. As one of the medical interns assigned to cover that floor, I was called in to examine patients who had a fever and any other bodily symptoms.

I remember one Dutch sailor who was so "schizophrenic" that I couldn't have gotten him to tell me his medical history even if I had spoken Dutch. But something about his wild ramblings — and his body temperature of 106°F — said "delirium" to me, and delirium in turn said "brain problem, possible infection." The stiffness of his neck and spine that I observed as two hefty orderlies "persuaded" him to lie curled up on his side for a spinal tap had already suggested meningitis, but I was nonetheless shocked when a geyser of pus sprayed out, just missing my left ear, as I pricked his spine with a needle.

Microscopic examination of the spinal fluid revealed that the cause of the Dutch sailor's psychosis was a microorganism, a bacterium, a "bug." And because the bacterium succumbed to penicillin, he was quickly and dramatically cured of both his meningitis and his delirium. During the balance of that mad, mad year, I saw many other patients whose brains were bugged, including one patient whose "paranoia" was caused by a tuberculosis abscess of his brain, and another whose "mania" was caused by a bacterial blockage of his blood vessels due to a heart infection.

There were scores of other patients, all of whom were said to have mental illnesses that, when unmasked, were the result of brain diseases. Many human problems are caused by brain abnormalities masquerading as mental illness. Any abnormal or exceptional mental state is a reflection of an abnormal or exceptional brain state. This book takes that idea very seriously.

Stop to consider the idea for just a second. It seems obvious, in retrospect, that my Dutch sailor's ranting and raving was caused by a brain disease (in 1960 physicians simply labeled him "crazy"). But there are thousands of other mental patients who rant and rave who have no known disease. There are hundreds of thousands more who have less dramatic but troublesome problems like anxiety, depression, and neurosis. Society readily assumes that all these people must have some history of psychological stress or trauma that has caused them to be this way. I say no. They rant and rave, or flit about nervously, or fail to show up for work, or carry Valium in their purses because there is a functional disorder of the state of their brain-mind. They may well have been abused as children, or have lost their self-esteem, and this can cause real emotional stress. But it does not cause the actual anxiety, depression, neurosis, or any other of a long list of problems. These problems are all caused by subtle physiological changes in the state of the brain-mind.

The idea works in reverse, too. There is no mystery about people who can hypnotize themselves, enter a trance, or meditate. While they may ascribe their ability to Buddhism, to mind control, or to concentration on the energy of the spirits around them, none of these practices actually causes them to shift gears unless they effect a change in brain-mind state. You can do all these things, too, without ever reading a word of Eastern philosophy or believing in magic or witchcraft.

WHAT IS THE MIND?

Until the nineteenth century most definitions of the mind were comfortably restricted to self-awareness. For most theorists, "consciousness" was akin to the ancient concept of spirit — a sentient form of energy that vitalized the body and moved it. Because of its link to the notion of a soul, this concept conceived the mind to be quite different from the brain and even separable from it.

Separability of mind from brain has also been an important aspect of religious philosophies that hold that the spirit may both antedate the body and survive it after death. For early Christian philosophers the doctrine of separability was tied to the primacy of God's will as the first, last, and ultimate cause of all things.

Even with the rise of mechanistic thinking in the Renaissance, the separability of brain and mind was maintained. In one variation of the French philosopher René Descartes's dualistic theory, separability was achieved by assuming that the brain and the mind were two perfectly synchronized mechanisms. According to Descartes, my awakening in Ogunquit involved simultaneous state changes of my brain and my mind, which reflected a perfect preordination of two parallel clocklike processes that were designed, wound up, and set ticking by God before I was born! Today this elaborate intellectual contrivance seems so strained as to be untenable to most modern thinkers. And yet, many of us still remain subtly but strongly committed to one or another form of dualism. How can we explain this paradox? What is the source of our deep resistance to the compelling idea of brain-mind unity?

The delirium of my dream may offer a clue, since it indicates that consciousness, invaluable and precious a tool though it may be, is a very poor judge of itself. It is often hopeless in correctly identifying its own state. To wit: I was dreaming but was convinced I was awake. Even when I am awake, it is difficult for me to imagine that my consciousness is a physical state of my brain.

The fact is that the huge knot of nerves in our heads has no nerve devoted to monitoring itself. We thus have no direct sensation of actually possessing a brain. We have to take it on faith. And while it is an idea that we all accept as anatomical truth, it almost never enters our consciousness as we think. Thus our philosophies have almost entirely ignored our brains.

You might suppose that the existence of headaches proves this idea to be wrong, but the nerve fibers that convey these painful impulses are in the walls of the blood vessels that supply the brain with its critical quotient of oxygen; they are not sensitive to the state of the brain itself.

Only some other part of consciousness, the faculty that we call self-awareness, is capable of observing our brain states. We say, "I'm getting quite forgetful in my old age," implying senility, or "My attention is flagging. I must need a good night's sleep," implying brain fatigue.

Vernacular expressions regarding incompetence or mental illness also refer to the brain-mind connection. Consider: "pea-brain" for someone who is not too bright; "bats in the belfry" for someone who is behaving oddly; "brainwashed" for the victims of cult conversion. But mostly we just don't think of ourselves, our thoughts, and our feelings as brain functions. It requires too much of a leap. And there is so much riding on it. Who wants to gamble and lose his immortality? But if I am right about brain-mind unity, then my mind, my being, will die with my brain. It will not fly off somewhere to another dimension in space and time.

My main point here, however, is not to challenge your belief about God or your soul. I am attempting to describe with scientific rigor how the brain-mind works while you are on this earth, regardless of whether you think a God put you here or that you have a soul that will carry on after you are dead.

BRAIN-MIND UNITY

The explosion of knowledge about physiology that began in the late nineteenth century first prompted the conviction of many scientists that brain and mind are one. That's why so many turn-of-the-century psychologists, including Sigmund Freud and William James, tried to formulate a unified brain-mind theory. The failure of these early efforts stemmed from the inability of the scientists to fit new, objective information about the brain to the subjective experience of the mind. However clearly relevant were the discoveries of brain electrical activity, brain cells, and brain molecules, it was impossible to see how the grand mental whole emerged from these tiny physical parts.

Although this difficulty led Freud and others to abandon the search for a brain-mind connection, evidence has steadily mounted over time to support it. The first major insight was the recognition that changes in the electrical activity of the brain correlated with sleep and awake states. This implied that consciousness had a definite and essential physical basis. Today, with sophisticated imaging technology, it is possible to observe these electrical changes in real time. Researchers can now project an image of my brain onto a computer screen as I sleep and show the changing electrical activity that occurs while I dream and when I wake up.

A second important insight was the discovery that each nerve cell in the brain — each neuron — is an independent electric-signal generator. Each neuron is capable of converting the metabolic energy derived from sugar and oxygen into electrical energy and of deploying an electrical charge to signal its own state of excitement to its neighbors. This gave rise to the idea that the brain could not only produce its own electrical energy but could use the rapid changes in energy level to encode information. The pattern of electrical signals arising in neurons could thus be conceived of as a sort of Morse code that could represent the external world within the brain (perception) and could go on to perform calculations on those representations (thinking, or cognition). Once the idea of representation via electrically coded signals was accepted, emotions, memories, and all the exquisite and tortured states of our conscious existence could begin to be modeled in physical terms.

A third seminal revelation was the appreciation that neuronal signaling was chemical as well as electrical. At the junction (or synapse) between any two neurons, the electrical state of one is communicated to the other via the release of chemical molecules called neurotransmitters. These chemicals are manufactured by the neurons themselves.

I no longer have any doubt that every detail of my Ogunquit dream can be accounted for in terms of neuronal signal patterns. My dream was just one of an infinite number of possible sets of self-generated brain signals. My brain generated the images, then concocted a story line to link them. Of course, the representations of the physical world stored in my gray matter, my personal history, and my emotional makeup all played an important role in the creation of the dream plot. For me, reducing the content of the dream to its representation in neuron signals robs the dream of none of its drama or significance. But even the drama and its significance are physically instantiated processes.

Utilizing the building blocks now available in the brain sciences, it is possible for us to understand how our conscious states are elaborated. Thought, memory, and emotion are realized in brain-cell activity patterns. And the brain cells are organized in such a way as to continuously shift from one activity pattern to another. The most dramatic and global shifts occur when we fall asleep, dream, and wake up. In these major states, and at the interfaces between them, the unity of the brain-mind reveals itself with startling clarity. That is why the states are the foundation of the unified theory.

FROM WAKING TO DREAMING . . . AND BACK AGAIN

The strongest evidence of brain-mind unity emerges day by day and night by night from the scientific study of waking, dreaming, and the stretches of sleep during which we may think or imagine but don't vividly dream. Over the past forty years, it has become clear that our brain-minds regularly alternate between two extremes when consciousness is at a peak — waking and dreaming. When we are awake our brain-minds are in the grip of one chemical system, and when we are dreaming our brain-minds are in the grip of a completely different chemical system. When both systems are at half-throttle, we sleep deeply with no dreams and little or no conscious mental activity.

The brain's chemical system that mediates our waking state is called the aminergic system. The molecules that do the work are amines. The chemical system that mediates dreaming is called the cholinergic system. Its molecule is acetylcholine. The two chemical systems are in dynamic equilibrium. This means — as we already know — that our conscious states fluctuate constantly and gradually between the extremes of waking and dreaming. Even at the extremes, both the aminergic (waking) and the cholinergic (dreaming) systems are active. Their predominance is only relative, not absolute. Thus, the two extreme states have shared as well as differentiated properties, at both the cellular-molecular and the experimental levels. Between the extremes is a rich continuum of aminergic-cholinergic interactions and an equally rich continuum of brain-mind states.

Some of the most interesting points along the continuum, such as fantasy, hypnosis, and meditation, have already begun to be elucidated in terms of the unified brain-mind state theory. The theory also enables us to understand less appealing altered states such as delirium, dementia, depression, and coma in a new and integrated way. And since our brain-mind theory is specified at the molecular level, chemical treatment of these unwanted states can be rationally prescribed. I will explore all these states and the means for altering them as this book moves ahead.

The greatest value of the brain-mind state concept is that it addresses the experience of waking, sleeping, and dreaming in a holistic way. Given the many microscopic details of brain science, it is possible for our conscious states to be integral only if the brain-mind operates according to a set of global physical-chemical conditions. And this, as you will see, is exactly what the aminergic-cholinergic control system guarantees via its widespread connections throughout the nervous system.

We need also to be able to account for the almost instantaneous changes from one conscious state to another. How, for example, is my conversion from the wild world of my New Orleans hotel dream to my awareness of a rainy Monday Ogunquit morning accomplished so seamlessly and efficiently? Within small parts of a second my brain-mind shifts from one self-consistent state (dreaming) to another (waking). To account for such a dramatic transition, we must discover a strongly centralized and highly hierarchical control system within the brain. The aminergic-cholinergic system is just that. From its strategic position at the base of the brain, it can command the state of the upper brain (where our thoughts and feelings are represented) at the same time that it controls the lower brain (which conveys sensations from our bodies and enacts our volition through muscular action). This switching system is as reliable as it is flexible. It is about as rare for me to gain awareness that I am dreaming when I am dreaming as it is for me to begin to hallucinate when I am awake.

The discreteness of conscious states so extreme as waking and dreaming must therefore be determined by the capacity of the aminergic-cholinergic control system to undergo very rapid switching. When I woke up in Ogunquit, the hotel dream scenario was immediately canceled as my aminergic wake-state system quenched my cholinergic dream-state system. This is possible because the brain cells deliver their electrochemical messages so quickly.

The brain-mind states are all the more wondrous when we appreciate just how different they are. In my dream I was entirely in the thrall of an internally generated scenario; a second later my state was replaced by a faithful representation of the external world. In a flash my feelings switched from acute panic to amused calm.

One inescapable upshot is that all the faculties of what we have heretofore called the mind (such as perception, orientation, emotion, and memory) operate in a consistent and unified way within each state. The other is that the instantiation of all those faculties in brain-signal processes is likewise consistent and unified. The conclusion is that brain-mind states are every bit as much functional *units* as are the neurons and neurotransmitters that mediate them. And likewise, our brain-mind states are encoded and can be accessed just like the phone numbers that are encoded as memories, or the terror and bliss that are encoded as emotions.

Brain-mind states are units of reality. If we can understand how they work we will be enormously empowered, because brain-mind states are not always adaptive or pleasant, and the knowledge will enable us to design more effective interventions for what we have always called "mental illness." It might well be more appropriate to label such unwanted conditions dysfunctional brain-mind states.

A CALM IN THE STORM

One of the most obvious applications for our new understanding of brain-mind states is in sleep science, which is expanding rapidly. Sleep disorders, sleep labs, and sleep centers are springing up everywhere. Gone forever is the myth of sleep as simple, benign, and uneventful. At last there is some balm for the anguish of the night.

Every day, new phenomena are described: adults stop breathing only to gasp for air; babies stop breathing in their cribs and die; men dive off beds into dream swimming pools or tackle bureau drawers in dream football games; others shake, rattle, and roll (and even kick) their sweet wives. Depressives awaken unrefreshed and are given drugs to prevent them from dreaming; then they wake up with renewed vigor.

What is going on here? What can the brain-mind paradigm tell us about all of this? For starters, it tells us that we are lucky there is not more disorder in our lives. At a deeper level, it tells us that much of the disorder is understandable and controllable — using the simplifying assumptions of the brain-mind theory.

CHAPTER 2

Brain-Mind Schizophrenia

I WAS ANGRY. I knew I had to go there, but I did not want to. I walked down the long white hallway, slowly, until I reached the open doorway on my right. I looked into the office. He was there. The man in the white coat. Was he Jesus Christ? Or God? I had been in this building before. It was a house of peace and rest. But I knew better than to go into his office. I knelt at the doorway, genuflected, and said, "I am a good Catholic." The man inside the office walked toward me. I looked up at him as he approached. I was tense. I lunged at him, my fists clenched, but he slipped out of the way. I turned and stared angrily at him. He said, "Your feelings are normal and healthy, even though they are confused and out of control."

ANOTHER ONE of my odd dreams? Not at all. It happened to a man I know named Bertal. But for him it wasn't a dream. He was wide awake when he hallucinated it and acted it out. The building he was in was a mental hospital in Boston. He was a patient. I was his doctor — the man in the white coat. And he lunged at me with so much force I was only lucky to dodge his assault.

Bertal's waking experience certainly seems like a dream experience, doesn't it? And it is, in an important way: the image of the house of peace, and of Jesus, was as real to Bertal as the New Orleans hotel and gun-toting guard had been to me. Three minutes before I woke up from my dream in Ogunquit, I was as crazy as Bertal. My dreaming was a conscious brain-mind state. Bertal's hallucinations and delusions were a conscious brain-mind state. Only for me, the state occurred when I was asleep, as it should have. For Bertal, it occurred when he was awake, when it shouldn't have. Mental illnesses, I maintain, are disordered brain-mind states.

I vividly remember the day I met Bertal. He was the first patient of my residency in psychiatry at the Massachusetts Mental Health Center in Boston. Like Bellevue in New York City, the place had informally been dubbed The Psycho. It seems that people everywhere call mental hospitals by nicknames that capture our collective ignorance — and fear — of being out of our minds.

I was relieved to have completed my Bellevue internship without contracting tuberculosis, as three of my eleven colleagues had, without being assaulted or even murdered by a psychotic patient, as also sometimes happened, and without suffering from that most pernicious disease of doctors — cynical detachment. Instead, I was full of hope and excitement as I drove to Boston in the early morning light of July 1, 1960. I was still in my hospital whites because I had stayed up all night successfully treating a young woman in diabetic coma. It seemed like a fitting and satisfying end to one chapter of my life, and I was eager to begin the new one: my education in real psychiatry, real mental illness, not just the brain disease I had seen at Bellevue.

Mass. Mental was indeed a temple of hope. It was the dawn of the 1960s, and not just psychosis and neurosis but all the social problems of mankind were deemed mental illnesses in the sense that they were viewed as learned behaviors that could be unlearned and reversed via psychoanalysis. Like many other young people, I was out to save the world.

Bertal was a twenty-three-year-old electronics worker who had been admitted about this time of year during each of the prior two years. His mother brought him in each time, and this summer she had told the staff that Bertal had been under pressure following a recent job promotion. He had fully withdrawn from communicating in the last two days. Doctors at The Psycho thought Bertal's mental illness was caused by his mother's overprotective behavior. They thought she was so psychologically toxic that they labeled her "schizophrenogenic." Bertal's psychotic confusion, they said, was a reaction to his mother's mixed signals.

I must confess that although I wondered a bit about the plausibility of this notion, I tended to accept it because my august mentors said it was so. And I suppose some part of me wanted to believe it, too. Because if this "bad mother" theory was correct, all we would need to do was separate Bertal from his toxic parent and cure him with clear communication signals. At our planning meeting, not one word was mentioned to me about the brain, about neurotransmitters, or about the possibility of a chemical genesis or remedy for Bertal's problem.

When I first met Bertal (a few weeks before the lunging incident), he looked physically healthy, well-built, and neatly dressed. But he was incredibly anxious, shifting from one foot to the other, wringing his hands, and staring at the ceiling of my office. His vocabulary was usually limited to guttural grunts, so he surprised me when he once suddenly said, "I should have went swimming."

The next day the orderlies had to forcibly restrain Bertal to keep him in the ward. He was extremely withdrawn and angry. We telephoned his mother and she came in. In seeming confirmation of the bad mother idea, she was very protective and dominant toward him. In her presence, Bertal became tearful and clinging, and he begged her to take him home.

My conversations with Bertal in subsequent sessions went nowhere. He fluctuated from being aloof or apologetic to being angry or violent. A senior psychoanalyst at The Psycho told me I should not give medication to Bertal even during his worst episodes. He said that even though Bertal was a massively anxious and grossly psychotic young man, medication constituted a chemical straitjacket that would damage his ability to enter into a psychotherapeutic relationship with me. Our "relationship" soon became ridiculous. As Bertal hallucinated an end-of-the-world bombing and strafing raid, I was trying to coax him to enter my office to discuss his feelings about his mother. When, in mortal terror of the dive-bombers, he ran out of the hospital and crawled under a parked car, I ran after him, lay down on the curbstone, and performed a wild sort of sidewalk psychoanalysis. Later, when Bertal was in the grips of an even more terrifying waking nightmare, my psychoanalyst supervisor made the mistake of entering the seclusion room where the orderlies had put Bertal for his own protection. Bertal mistook him for the enemy and beat him up. The orderlies wrestled Bertal to the ground and put him on heavy doses of chlorpromazine — a tranquilizer.

Within a few days Bertal was sitting in my office, calm and collected, talking about his mother. He remained this way as long as he was on the medication.

Bertal's psychosis was the result of a spontaneous and cataclysmic brain-mind state change. Although we brain researchers don't yet know where such psychoses originate, we do know that Bertal's brain-mind state was converted from psychotic to nonpsychotic by a chemical process. What we also know now (but did not know then, unfortunately) is that chlorpromazine interacts with brain neurotransmitters so strongly that it was able to bamboozle Bertal's neurons into more stable behavior.

My experience with patients like Bertal forced me to be more skeptical of the adequacy of psychoanalysis. Second, it forced me to consider how those two most difficult of medical school subjects, physiology and biochemistry, might be helpful in constructing a more adequate theory of mental-state change than was possible using psychology alone. This is because Bertal's psychosis was undoubtedly mediated by chemicals within the brain, regardless of whether it had anything to do with his psychological conflict with his mother. Even if psychoanalysis ultimately proved useful in understanding Bertal, it was clearly not as good as chemistry in restoring normal functioning to his psychotic brain-mind.

But how in the world were we to account for the efficacy of a chemical? At the time, we knew that chlorpromazine was an antihistamine. Its tranquilizing effects had been discovered by accident as it was being tried out as a cold remedy! We did not know, however, why it cleared Bertal's mind of dive-bomber hallucinations.

Today we know that chlorpromazine blocks the action of at least one neurotransmitter. But we do not understand exactly why that helps. In the absence of a full explanation we are still in the dark about psychosis. Even though we may take some satisfaction in being able to alter such states chemically, we can't be content without a more adequate theory of normal and abnormal mental states, one that is built up from the physiology of the brain. That theory — the brain-mind state theory — is the central subject of this book. Because the theory sets forth a specific model of how conscious states develop, I call that model the brain-mind paradigm.

There is an important experimental point to realize here, too. Just as the visual images of my hotel dream were entirely fabricated by my brain, so Bertal's religious delusions were fabricated by his brain. This recognition radically alters our understanding of psychosis. There is no way for us to regard Bertal's dive-bomber hallucinations as essentially different from our own dream projections. We can therefore regard our own dreams as a proper basis for studying a normal process that becomes exaggerated in psychosis; projective perception escapes its confinement to one state — dreaming — and invades another — waking. This is why I base the brain-mind paradigm on the study of states and especially conscious states like dreaming.

FREUD VERSUS SKINNER: THEY'RE BOTH WRONG

Before discussing the brain-mind paradigm, it will help us to recognize the conflict that has raged for ninety years between neurology (the study of the brain) and psychology (the study of the mind), for the context and foundation of the new paradigm springs from this conflict. Inspired by the rapid growth of neuroscience, these two fields have recently evolved in the direction of brain-mind integration. There is finally a groundswell, a coalescing of ideas.

In 1890 a clear concept of brain-mind unity was laid out by American philosopher and psychologist William James in *The Principles of Psychology*. James carefully presented a comprehensive vision of what happens inside our heads. He tried to integrate the then-current theories about the brain with those emerging from observations of people made during psychology experiments. In Vienna, Sigmund Freud was trying to do exactly the same thing at exactly the same time. But James and Freud simply did not know enough about the physical brain to make it work. Although James stuck with it, Freud abandoned this early goal of building up clinical psychology from brain science.

By 1920 neurology had begun to fade into the background, while psychology had grown. But psychology itself was undergoing a civil war, led by two of the greatest intellectual adventurers of the twentieth century: Sigmund Freud, the father of psychoanalysis, and B. F. Skinner, the father of behaviorism. Freud held that our actions were rooted in deep dark impulses, particularly those that had to do with sex, which were stored in our unconscious minds. These motivated our conscious behavior. He maintained that these impulses "got out" of the unconscious when we were asleep, and caused dreams. Thus, the study of dreaming became the province of psychoanalysts. To Freud, neurology was good only for explaining body processes, such as eating or walking. (Freud also feared that lending any credence to neurology would weaken his new theory and his burgeoning psychoanalytic movement.)

Skinner and the behaviorists went even further. They, too, ignored the brain, calling it a "black box." But they were also disdainful of the introspective experience that interested Freud and the psychoanalysts; to the behaviorists, only outwardly observable motor acts were suitable data for a scientific psychology. All behavior was learned, and all actions were reactions to stimuli.

As a consequence, neurology and psychology proceeded along two parallel but completely separate paths for well over half a century. Among the many victims of the divergence was medicine, and especially psychiatry. Although psychiatry was born a hybrid of neurology and psychology, it vacillated between the two (as my experience with Bertal proved) and led young doctors like me to try to talk to patients under cars one day and inject them with chlorpromazine the next. Ironically and sadly, psychiatry had become increasingly distant from brain science at precisely the time when psychiatry had so much to gain from it. Within psychiatry, confusion reigned supreme; there were therapists who were sensitive to patients' psychological conflicts and reluctant to prescribe pills, and others who prescribed medication freely but were often insensitive to the personal concerns of their patients.

THE NEW NEUROSCIENCE

This clinical turmoil still persists today, and clearly it is still as undesirable as it is unacceptable. Psychoanalysts and behaviorists have all failed to offer definitive or lasting solutions to the problem of psychosis. And many of the drugs of psychiatrists, such as Valium, Tegretol, and Clozaril, while dramatically powerful, are still problematic because they cannot be targeted to specific brain systems; in most cases we don't even know which brain systems to target! All this makes the conscientious physician unhappy. We need the conceptual and experimental tools with which to do better. Thankfully, they are now being forged in the brain-mind workshops of the world.

A basic concept we need is one that explains the natural relationship between brain-mind disorder and order. For this we turn to the emerging theories about chaos. Mathematicians and physicists, like my colleague David Kahn, tell us that all complex systems — and the brain-mind is a very complex system — have intrinsically chaotic properties. The brain-mind is thus like the weather; knowing its state today does not allow us precisely to predict its state tomorrow. Thus we must accept ourselves as, to a degree, unpredictable.

Chaos theory maintains, however, that the unpredictability is balanced by an equally intrinsic capacity for self-organization. From self-organization arises an emergent order that may be as unanticipated as the chaos that gave rise to it. Human creativity depends on a natural tension between the chaos and the self-organization of brain-mind states. Dreaming is indeed a chaotic brain-mind state, yet it has long been celebrated by many artists who tap their dreams as sources of inspiration, such as the English poet Samuel Taylor Coleridge, who wrote "Kubla Khan," the Spanish surrealist Salvador Dali, who painted *The Persistence of Memory*, and Robert Louis Stevenson, author of *The Strange Case of Dr. Jekyll* (order) *and Mr. Hyde* (chaos).

But mathematical models are not enough. People want to see physical evidence that there is order in the chaos of the brain. The evidence is found in the neuroscience labs of the world, which are monitoring the brain activity of everyone from sleeping college students to Alzheimer's patients. It is now possible in the sleep lab that I run for Harvard Medical School at the Massachusetts Mental Health Center, for example, to watch the brain at work each night. And by using new imaging technology that transmits images of the brain's electrical activity onto a computer screen, we may see that the same visual area of my brain lights up when I see a real gun pointed at me or when I dream of a security guard drawing a bead on my head or even when I voluntarily conjure up an image of a gun in my mind's eye. It would also be possible, today, to see if Bertal's dive-bombers are his experience of hot spots in the visual part of his brain. If you live another decade, you yourself may well see all these things on the local news shows and in magazines, as more living, thinking, feeling, and dreaming brains are placed under positron-emission tomography scanners, magnetic resonance imagers, and magnetoencephalograms.

This new field of brain-mind study, called cognitive neuroscience, is the joyous second marriage of neurology and psychology after nearly a century of cold estrangement. Rejuvenated psychologists have found their way back to the study of consciousness by applying behaviorist methods to the study of such mental faculties as perception, memory, and emotion (instead of limiting themselves to Freud's scandalous unconscious). And today's neurologists are like children at Christmas; with so many new toys for playing brain games, they're lining up awaiting their turns. The kids who get to play first are the cognitive neuroscientists, the brain-mind people. Thanks to their efforts, we can begin to sketch the new brain-mind paradigm.

PRINCIPLES OF THE BRAIN-MIND PARADIGM

Three fundamental principles make up the brain-mind paradigm. The first is that the brain-mind is a unified system. The brain and mind are inextricably linked: no brain, no mind. Furthermore, when I dream of criminals in a hotel and when Bertal hallucinates dive-bombers, our respective brain-minds have entered states that have common physiological and psychological traits. We can use physiology to predict psychology, and psychology to predict physiology. That is, if we are "seeing things," it is likely that our visual brain is activated. Conversely, if our visual brain is activated, it is likely we are "seeing things." Three bold corollaries of this unification principle hold: that consciousness is the brain's awareness of its own physical state; that consciousness is a tool for studying the brain; and that consciousness is a tool for changing brain activity in strategic and healthful ways.

The second fundamental principle of the brain-mind paradigm is that there are three cardinal brain-mind states: waking, sleeping, and dreaming. These are the fundamental organizational units of the brain-mind. It may even be asserted that they are the highest level of organization of the brain-mind because they determine, in a powerful and reliable way, the quality and quantity of our experience. There are many other brain-mind states, such as drunkenness, sleepwalking, and coma, but in comparison these prevail during only short intervals. It follows that the more we can learn about how the three cardinal brain-mind states are organized, the more we can understand conscious experience and the way in which consciousness can alter, for good or bad, brain-mind states. My hotel dream and Bertal's war psychosis are variants of the same organizational unit: I don't know I'm dreaming, and he doesn't know he is psychotic. Both of us are completely convinced that we are awake, seeing the real world, and feeling threatened.

The third principle is that brain-mind states can be measured and manipulated, and thus understood. We have already seen that brain-mind states are controlled by a brain-within-the-brain, the aminergic-cholinergic system. This chemical system provides a solid link between neurology, psychology, and the psychiatric use of drugs. And researchers are learning so much more each day that we can already perceive an extension of our knowledge into less understood but important brain-mind states, such as psychosis, depression, and hypnosis.

For Bertal to hallucinate while awake and for me to hallucinate while asleep, some common shift in the balance of our brain chemical state-control systems must occur. By learning what happens in my brain-mind, we can gain insight into what happens in his. By illuminating the specific chemistry of shifts in the control system, we can then fully understand the favorable effect of chemicals on Bertal's hallucinations, thereby not merely relieving him of his fear, but enlightening him to his problem and how to control it.

If these claims are even partially true, then the new paradigm is worthy of our respectful and excited attention. I suspect that it is far truer even than it now appears.

COMPUTERS, GALAXIES, AND THE BUDDHA

As we move ahead on this journey of discovery, it is comforting to know we don't go it alone. New ideas bearing fruit in other areas of science and the humanities are helping us refine our model. Computer scientists, for example, have successfully built computers that exhibit so-called artificial intelligence. These are systems that process data over and over, and as they do so, they discern patterns within the data. The patterns are automatically entered into the software that runs the computer, which alters how the computer responds to new data. The computer refines its responses by running small test programs on itself. This is a useful way to think about how we ourselves learn. The neurons in our heads store data and perceive patterns. One theory about dreams is they are the test programs, which we initiate during our sleep to test our responses. In the computer science model, our dreams are diagnostics that we create during sleep to make sure our processors stay sharp.

From sleep research we learn that our brains continuously process information, even while we are in the deepest sleep. Until recently it was thought that the brain-mind required external stimuli to keep it going. Big names in psychology, including Ivan Pavlov, who taught dogs to salivate at the ringing of a bell, mistakenly believed that our brains shut off at night like the lights in our bedrooms. Even today there are popular notions that the stimulus that triggers a dream when we are asleep is external, be it a truck driving past our window, an experience we had during the day, or even indigestion. But we now see in sleep labs that no external stimulus is necessary or even sufficient to induce dreaming. Most nerve cells in the brain fire all the time, all day and all night. Our brain-minds do not merely react. They anticipate. They generate their own images. And they do so spontaneously, continuously, and automatically.

This is fortunate! Suppose we had to remember to breathe? One moment of forgetfulness and we'd all be dead. We are not, however, only automata whose central processors keep clicking away. While we do enjoy some of the reliability of a robot, we also are free to choose what goes into our minds and bodies. The information we choose to process, and the food and drugs we choose (or not) to take, influence our brain-mind states. As such, the brain-mind paradigm gives us not only the freedom of choice but also the burden of responsibility.

We have more to learn. Brain scientists now tell us there are on the order of 100 billion neurons in our brains, that each one may contact 10,000 others, and that each can send up to 100 messages a second. Modest estimates of the total information processing are upward of 10^{27} bits of data a second. That's 1,000,000,000,000,000,000,000,000,000 bits. It is easy to visualize the brain-mind as a roiling cauldron of witch's brew about to boil over. It seems bound to go haywire. And at times, for people like Bertal, it does.

Why don't we all have flights of manic psychosis or episodes of epilepsy? We're not certain. But we do know that a major result of the tension between the aminergic and cholinergic systems is the chemical restraint of our complex brain-mind system. Galaxies have orderly solar systems, oceans have dependable currents, weather has the steady trade winds. Brain-mind states self-organize, too, and are helped to do so by the aminergic-cholinergic system. Our brain-minds can and do occasionally jump out of this equilibrium. Some people go insane. The rest of us just dream — or change our minds. These events are the supernovas, tidal waves, and thunderstorms of our lives.

We learn even from Eastern philosophy. Buddhists view consciousness as causal, even in a physiological sense. They practice meditation not only for peace of mind but also to heal the body. Change the state of the mind and you can change the state of the body. We in the West are beginning to embrace this idea, as more stories surface of people who have staved off cancer or other ills by positive thinking and sheer will to survive.

WHY A NEW PARADIGM?

As I advance the new brain-mind theory here, I will try to shed light on some of the most perplexing questions of our existence. Why do we need sleep? How do we learn? What happens to our brain-minds as we age? Since we all seem to struggle with an attention deficit disorder after poor sleep, I hint that one function of sleep may be to reduce the probability of disorder inherent in such a spring-loaded machine as our brain-mind.

Another thorny issue to confront is that old demon determinism. It led Freud to erroneously assume that the brain-mind was doomed to fatally reenact conflicted scenarios. The brain-mind paradigm recognizes the reality of determinism, but it maintains that the system is too noisy simply to repeat itself. It is constantly being jostled into new states. Certainly the states can recur, as they do during the recurring dreams suffered by Vietnam vets. But I will go so far as to suggest that no two brain-mind states are ever perfectly identical.

One guarantee of state diversity is the passage of time. Because our brains and personal histories are changing at every second, we are never in exactly the same informational state twice. For better or worse, we need constantly to update our internal store of representations (call them memories if you like) to keep a running account of what is, after all, the perpetual novelty of the outside world.

How do we do it? If you are getting my message, you will have already guessed the answer: by the constant cycling of our brain-mind states, from waking to sleeping to dreaming. There is a time to collect data and a time to process it. This informational cycle is as automatic as breathing itself. We don't have to remember to do it. It just happens. Experiments to determine what, electrically and chemically, is occurring when we store new data and learn from it, even during sleep, are already in the works.

Psychiatry is in deep crisis. Psychoanalysis is clearly a cure-all that has failed, and drug-dependent psychiatry just as clearly has failed to become a cure-all. Into the breach we march. We desperately need a new brain-mind paradigm that will allow us to rescue the noble goals of psychoanalysis, tie them in a meaningful way to the strengths of pharmacology, and integrate the whole package with the burgeoning sciences of the brain and cognition.

This book attempts nothing less than such an integration. It does so by bringing together the most recent findings of modern research on waking, sleeping, and dreaming. The new brain-mind paradigm is as bold as it is modest. It is bold in that it aspires to comprehensiveness. And it is modest in recognizing that it is still incomplete. If you can stand such ambition of ends in the face of such humility of means, I welcome you to give yourself to this endeavor.

CHAPTER 3

Delia's Dream Delirium

TO PROVIDE a deeper description of what brain-mind states are, I will examine one exceptional example that happens to be well known to us all: dreaming. Dreaming is the state scientists can best analyze and diagnose today. Oddly enough, scientists have spent little time actually analyzing our brain activity when we are awake, but there is a volume of data on dreaming. Once my analysis is done, dreaming will become a touchstone for the other brain-mind states that I will discuss as this book progresses.

Mental states have traditionally been assessed by neurologists and psychiatrists using a question-and-answer format called the mental status exam. The mental status exam was conceived in the late 1800s and was an integral part of the clinical examination of a new patient. The central idea of the exam was that organic disease of the brain could be revealed through noticeable defects in memory, orientation, perception, and language, whether or not the patient showed any specific signs of neurological damage in the physical exam. In particular, some forms of psychosis could be shown to be organic using only the mental status exam.

This useful tool fell through the clinical cracks when psychology and neurology diverged early in this century. Psychologists concentrated on a patient's emotional past while neurologists became preoccupied with hardware that could tweak the brain. Both neglected the mental status exam. Today we can resurrect and amplify the usefulness of the mental status exam using the tools of modern cognitive science.

Scientists interested in normal and abnormal states of the brain-mind have long focused on dreaming because it shares so many of the formal features of what we call mental illness. The intense visual images of our dreams are like the visual hallucinations that frequently occur in toxic states like the DTs. Our conviction as we dream that the physically impossible events we experience are real is like the delusional belief that is the hallmark of psychosis. The stories that we concoct to explain improbable and impossible dream events are like the confabulations of delirium. The intense anxiety we suffer during nightmares approaches that experienced by people with panic disorder. And the poor memory we have of dreams once we awaken from them is similar to the memory lapses experienced by Alzheimer's patients and people with other tragic forms of dementia.

Almost a century ago the Swiss psychiatrist Carl Jung said, "Let the dreamer awake and you will see psychosis." But what *kind* of psychosis did Jung expect to see when he examined dreaming? He never answered that question. Could our nightly madness be likened to the bizarre thinking and emotional dulling of schizophrenia? Or do we see the wild flights of mania or encounter the dolorous delusions of depression? Is dreaming most like the delirium of organic brain rot — the spoilage that occurs when people persistently pickle their brain cells in beer, wine, and pot? Or does dreaming resemble the dementia that occurs in older people as their neurons die away?

One reason that Jung never considered these questions is that he came under the influence of Freud, who was convinced that dreaming was "the royal road to the unconscious." Freud made his move to draft Jung into the psychoanalytic army just when Jung was making quantitative studies that showed that a loosening of associations was not only the most essential characteristic of dreams, but also that it was a key symptom of schizophrenia. Neither Jung nor Freud made the obvious move of performing a mental status exam on dreaming, their own model of mental illness. I think the reason is clear — they became so caught up in the analysis of the *content* of particular dreams that they lost sight of the *form* of all dreaming.

Having come to this conclusion several years ago, I decided to find out for myself: What *kind* of madness *is* dreaming? What sort of unconscious mental processes are revealed? And what is the point of going nuts four or five times every night of my life?

Let's analyze some dreams.

One of the great pleasures of working on sleep and dreaming is that everyone you meet has something interesting to tell you about his or her experience. Far from dreading being offended by these often wild and woolly dream reports, I relish them. And they come not only from friends, students, and family members but from dreamers the world over, many of whom share their remarkable dream diaries with me and my colleagues.

One such correspondent, a student of mine named Delia, was a particularly prolific dreamer and remarkably diligent dream journalist. She kindly lent me a copy of her dream manuscripts recorded between November 29, 1988, and June 30, 1992, a treasure trove of 1,001 nights. From this I have selected several typical examples for this book. They are given verbatim, with Delia's permission, on condition only that I conceal the identities of the characters. In discussing the personal aspects of Delia's dreams I draw inferences from the reports themselves and from what I have learned from my relationship with Delia and others like her.

On April 19, 1989, Delia awakened and reported dreaming of being in a balloon over Paris and staying near the Al-Aqsa Mosque.

> I was with my sisters and father in a balloon over the city of Paris. There were other balloonists in the air as well. The view of the city was spectacular, and we were watching a golf tournament going on below. We were having a problem keeping the balloon steady in the wind, and kept bobbing up and down and were even coming close to some power lines. So my father and sisters decided to

change our plans — which called for our arriving back in the United States later that same day — in favor of landing and spending the night in Paris.

So we landed. As I got out of the basket, I thought to myself, Well, here I am standing in Paris for the first time! I followed my family through a beautiful public garden and down to the seashore (Paris was on the North Sea in my dream). There we took our shoes off to wade out into the water. I noticed, however, a large tanker off shore, and saw a young boy peeing in the water, so I wondered how badly the water was polluted as I stepped back out.

We walked to a large, old hotel next to the garden to get a room. I assumed it would be rather expensive since it was such a fancy place. I caught a glimpse of Al-Aqsa Mosque across the street from the hotel, so I asked the woman behind the desk about it. She pointed it out on a map. The mosque and connected buildings (some 28 in number) took up a full block in the city. I asked if the other buildings comprised an Islamic university, but she couldn't answer me since no one had asked about the mosque before.

As I looked at the map, it seemed to become a live aerial view of the property. There were mattresses all around the open spaces between the buildings for the refugees. The lady behind the desk pointed out the entrance to the mosque on the map. I began to make plans to get up early to say my morning prayers there.

In this long dream sequence there are four distinct scenes: (1) flying in the balloon, (2) landing in Paris, (3) walking to the hotel, and (4) looking at the map.

Notice that Delia indulges her adventurous wanderlust in the company of important family members. Her father and two sisters are with her in the balloon. Despite the exhilaration of flying and the spectacular vantage point, there is obvious anxiety about the safety of the craft and they all decide against crossing the ocean in the balloon that night.

Deciding to land in Paris puts the high anxiety of scene one on the terra firma of scenes two and three without giving up all the exoticism of scene one. Delia has never been to Paris before. And this Paris is very special indeed. It is on the seaside, and the North Sea at that, and it harbors the Al-Aqsa Mosque (which is actually in Jerusalem).

Now the Freudian in us might say that this one, like all flying dreams, is a thinly concealed sexual wish. Delia has an incestuous desire for her father and "flying" with him allows this unacceptable wish to be first symbolized and then, ultimately, grounded. She will then sublimate her sexual desires in voyeuristic tourism. Seeing the boy urinating is evidence of this progressive displacement process and illustrates her guilt and fear of contamination by her unclean desires. Not yet clean enough, she ends up in church.

I must admit that these Oedipal speculations seem far-fetched and silly. And even if we were convinced that, through psychoanalysis, Delia could dredge up a forgotten trauma with her father, or uncover a repressed fear about a punitive mother, resulting in helpful clarification of sexual identity and choice-of-man issues, this interpretive approach overlooks something crucial. What is overlooked, and what is the window to analyzing Delia's dream state, is the *form* of her dreams. Studying the many formal features of her dream sequence could help us understand all dreams and the common brain-mind state that produces them in all of us.

Therefore I will perform a mental status exam. I will first look at the cognitive aspects of the dream — awareness, memory, sensory perception, and so on. Then I will examine the emotional aspects of the dream, such as anger or sorrow. Once I have performed the mental status exam on Delia's dreaming I can draw some strong conclusions about her brain-mind state and the kind of madness her dreaming represents. Here we go.

MENTAL STATUS EXAM

General Appearance and Behavior

Delia is an attractive blonde in her early thirties, neatly and fashionably dressed, with a shy, winsome smile, who speaks openly about her rich mental life. Although she is employed in a bank, she is psychologically minded and describes her philosophy as "definitely New Age." She is intelligent, curious, and seems to be an extremely reliable informant because the reports of her dream madness have great internal consistency. Delia says that dreaming occurs every night and although she is not always aware of it, she usually remembers at least two episodes, especially since she began keeping her bedside journal. In short, there is nothing in her waking appearance or behavior that would even faintly suggest psychosis.

Sensorium

Delia says that her consciousness during dreaming is usually unclouded: "as sharply clear as a Dali painting" is one of her phrases, "and equally strange." She says, for example, "The view of the city was spectacular, and we were watching a golf tournament going on below." She feels somewhat confused when she first snaps out of her dream state, but when in it, her mind is very attentive, although she usually has no awareness she is dreaming. For example, the four dream scenes she recorded flowed seamlessly in a single stream. So we conclude that her sensorium is clear.

Orientation

Delia is often a bit disoriented in her dreams; sometimes quite a lot. The people in her dreams are particularly fluid. Sometimes they don't look like the ones they are supposed to be, and sometimes they seem like two people, or even a hybrid of the two sexes. Sometimes characters appear out of nowhere; a woman suddenly becomes a man. Very often the identity of people is vague or uncertain.

Despite this uncertainty about other characters, Delia is sure she is herself and not someone else (like the Virgin Mary, Joan of Arc, or Josephine Bonaparte). Very rarely she sees herself as an actress on the stage of her dreams. But she almost always views the action from the center of her brain-mind. (Many people, myself included, never see themselves as a third person in their dreams.) Her first person, her "I," is always the same and is usually integral, while third persons, "they," are very commonly incongruous, ephemeral, or strangely constructed. But surprisingly, this orientation rarely seems bothersome to her.

Dream places are particularly likely to violate Aristotelian unity.

Dream objects are either out of place (like the Al-Aqsa Mosque and the seashore) or are internally inconsistent (like the mosque and its twenty-eight interconnected buildings). And we do not expect to see a boy urinating openly, even in Paris!

Time often jumps forward and backward, or is compressed or expanded. Who could expect to fly from Paris to the USA in one day in a balloon?

So, we need to underline *disorientation,* because Delia is obviously severely disoriented in her dreams.

Attention

When seized by a dream, the dreamer pays no attention to the outside world and makes no conscious selection of the internal data either. Delia didn't select what to look at; the scenes just appeared. Another thing she has also noticed is that she can't direct her thoughts as she normally can.

So we can conclude that Delia's brain-mind state of dreaming is characterized by a high degree of both *distractibility* and *absorption.* This dream feature is so common and so overwhelmingly strong that we usually don't even mention it. It combines with the disorientation of dreaming in an interesting way: we can now say that this particular brain-mind state is characterized by constant shifts in both the orienta*tion* sense (time, place, and person) and the orient*ing* sense (attentional direction).

Memory

Delia says her memory of her dreams is usually quite good. Compared with her friends, she has two or three times as much recall. The original report, 356 words, is not exceptionally long for her, but it is far above the fifty-word average of most people! Even so, Delia says she is sure that there are often many details she can't remember. Sometimes she is sure there have been previous episodes that cannot be recalled. And more often than not she will awaken unable to recall anything at all.

She is sometimes struck that surprisingly remote memories come back to her in her dreams. Equally striking are what Delia calls pseudo-memories, things that really never happened in real life. She says it is almost as if she fills in the blanks, makes it all up as she goes along. Delia knows quite a bit about this capacity of her brain-mind to confabulate. When memory fails her, she makes up for it with imagination.

And, indeed, these dreamy states of brain-mind do have a fabulous aspect. They are like fables, full of mystery, with mismatching features that nonetheless seem to fit.

So we have a third and fourth important finding to add to disorientation and attention deficit: *spotty recent memory* and its partner, *confabulation* (which patches up the story by filling in the holes). Delia already sounds a bit like my aunt Agatha, who got lost more and more frequently as she aged and then made up incredible stories to cover her tracks. She wasn't lying, she was just confabulating.

Intellectual Functions

Delia is an avid reader, but she shuns math and science. Interestingly, she rarely imagines reading any of these subjects when she is dreaming. She may spend her entire workday poring over papers or tables of numbers, but neither texts nor tables of any kind make an appearance in her dreams. We don't know whether she can read during her dreams or understand what she has read, whether she can subtract 7 from 100, or name the presidents back to JFK. It may not seem important, but the *lack* of this kind of content is also striking evidence of a difference in brain-mind states because it suggests a loss of that whole set of higher brain-mind skills we call rational analysis. Even professors, like me, never dream of reading or writing.

Language and Stream-of-Talk

Delia's dream lacks dialogue in situations that would seem to call for it. Nowhere in her report of three highly social scenarios is there an "I said"/"He said" sequence. In fact, there is no quotable language at all. She does not report the nervous conversation that would have been natural among herself, her father, and her sisters when the balloon was bobbing up and down near the power lines. They just decided to change their plans without discussing it. This is a typical dream feature: when conversation seems indicated, it is often only implied.

Upon landing, Delia does have a bit of a conversation with herself when she thinks, Well, here I am standing in Paris for the first time. But this isn't much of a conversation and it isn't even much of a thought, since it is a conclusion not supported by the data (witness the beach, the tanker, the peeing boy, and the mosque).

Mental Content

This category of the mental status exam has always struck me as ill-named because it doesn't deal with the content at all. Instead, it emphasizes the form in which activity is presented. The content of Delia's dream is expressed in the form of hallucinations (false perceptions) and delusions (false beliefs). The whole dream scenario, for that matter, is fictive.

The first aspect of the dream's mental form to consider is the richness of the visual and motor perceptions that are the main ground of Delia's dream experience. The people, places, and actions in her dream are all fully realized; they are not amorphous images or voices that come from offstage. She *hallucinates* them. Delia actually sees her father and two sisters in the balloon basket. She sees the golf tournament, the power lines, the beautiful public garden, the seashore, the tanker, the peeing boy, the Al-Aqsa Mosque, and the mattresses laid out for the refugees.

Two things are so obvious about all of this that they might escape notice. One is that the scene of the dream is constant and vivid; so is her sense of being in the scene and *moving through it*. The main hallucinatory aspect of the brain-mind state might then be characterized as visuomotor rather than as simply visual. (The term visuomotor captures the cinematic aspect of dreaming — the constantly changing scene and our perpetual movement through it.)

Although Dali's paintings are a suitable metaphor for the strange surrealistic quality of Delia's dream experience, they are *static,* whereas Delia's visions are not. Dali's famous surrealist film *The Andalusian Dog* is a more adequate metaphor, because both its vision and its motion are continuous. The silence of that film is also accurate in mimicking the relative weakness of the auditory sense during dreams, which I have already noted as the lack of clear speech. Weaker still are the sensations of touch, temperature, taste, and smell; none of these are present in Delia's account.

I emphasize the almost constant motion of Delia's dream because the illusion of movement is common to all dreams. In scene one Delia is struggling to steady the bobbing balloon. In scene two, she walks through the garden, takes off her shoes, and wades in the water before walking on to the hotel. These are all active, transitive movements of the dream body through the dream space.

Let's now consider the psychological aspects of the dream. It could, certainly, prompt psychoanalytic speculation. I have already pointed out the possibly Oedipal meaning of this balloon jaunt with daddy and shown how Delia's anxiety at being aloft with him might lead to the safety of their grounding. We have even admitted the possible import of the urination-pollution vision and concern. Nothing in my formal analysis contradicts these speculative ideas. I understand and acknowledge that parents are important, that they do powerfully shape psychosexual attitudes and behaviors. And without endorsing them as truth, I simply point out that all these "interpretations" reveal "meanings" that are already blatant and transparent in the dream.

When it comes to delusions, Delia's case becomes much more subtle. Are the misidentifications, such as this Paris-by-the-sea, the Paris with a mosque, really delusions? They are indeed. And the ability of Delia's father and sisters to change their mind and so descend the balloon is very much like the thought projection and related feelings of being mentally transparent that bother many people suffering from psychosis. There is no discussion among them, but it is as if her father and sisters knew she wanted to stop. So we can say, yes, *there are delusions,* and quite magical ones at that, but we note that the delusions are benign, not menacing. Delia does not imagine herself to be persecuted by the FBI, the Ku Klux Klan, or the mafia, those real-life demons that threaten our most psychotic brethren. So there is *no paranoia,* a crucial negative finding, since schizophrenia and bipolar affective disorder (two of the major brain-mind states that cause psychosis) are often loaded with paranoia.

Insight and Judgment

Let's consider insight first. It's just not there. Delia thinks she is awake even though the action that is going on could never occur in the waking state. How can she be so wrong about something so obvious? We marvel when we hear descriptions of what people — both sane and insane — ardently believe. But isn't it truly mind-boggling that with the many striking and distinctive signs of psychosis that are always present in the dream state, we almost never recognize it for what it is?

Jean-Paul Sartre, the French existentialist philosopher, asserted that lack of insight was the most distinctive feature of dreaming. He called it a "lack of self-reflective awareness." I like his point. The lack of self-monitoring, or what Sartre calls self-consciousness, prevents us from calling ourselves fool when we are caught, again and again, in a madhouse of our own devising.

In waking, we possess an almost uncanny capacity to track our thoughts and our behavior as they unfold. By means of self-monitoring we conduct a continuous negotiation between our own goals and social constraints, between our here-and-now ideas and our there-and-then hopes, between our cognitions and our feelings.

Delia does maintain a social conscience. Notice her accommodation of her family's concerns about danger in orchestrating the balloon's landing, her withdrawal from the urine-contaminated water, and her concern about the luxurious expense of the hotel.

But even with this ability to judge, Delia is *not aware of her true state of consciousness.* When she is awake she might say of her suspicions, "I wonder if I am getting paranoid," or of her momentary lapses when she may be absorbed in fantasy, "I must have been daydreaming." But almost never is Delia able to notice that she is dreaming while she is dreaming. And even if, for a fleeting instant, she were to say to herself, "This is so crazy that it must be a dream," her insight immediately leaves her and she is pulled back into delusion.

Emotion

There is more to dreaming than the various cognitive qualities charted above. There is the whole domain of feelings. Our feelings serve as a way to know the world that is completely different from thinking. Feelings can tell us about our states and those of others. We have powerful "first impressions" and often base important decisions on our "gut feeling." Yet in the West, emotion is contrasted with rational knowing; it is almost treated as a cognitive nuisance. It is as if we didn't want to acknowledge that emotions are just as valid a way to perceive the world around us as that provided by our senses and our thoughts.

Delia's feelings move from excitement, elation, and anxiety (in the balloon) to surprise and pleasure (in Paris) to disgust (in the pissy water). Thus there is a transition from hot to cool feelings in the first half of the dream.

So this part of Delia's mental status exam does not indicate any predominant emotion or type of emotions. Typically, the brain-mind state of dreaming has a majority of hot, or high-side, emotions (like anxiety, anger, or joy) and a minority of cool, or low-side, emotions (like sadness, shame, or remorse). Not only do the high-side emotions tend to occur more frequently, they are often more intense. This is especially true of fear and anxiety. But it is not uncommon to have balance, as Delia does.

In addition, Delia's dream emotions are always appropriately tied to her cognitive experiences. There is no separation of thoughts and feelings in dreaming, as occurs in schizophrenia. Her brain-mind state of dreaming, unlike schizophrenia, is not characterized by attenuated or suppressed feelings, and it is not characterized by either intolerably strong depressive feelings or by the giddy elation that disrupts cognition and judgment in mania.

In short, the emotional aspect of Delia's dream is natural and healthy.

DIAGNOSING DELIA'S DREAM: A CASE OF DELIRIUM

This examination of the cognitive domains of Delia's dreaming brain-mind has revealed several striking features: disorientation; distractibility; spotty memory and confabulations; visuomotor hallucinations and delusions; and a lack of insight that appears to be related to a loss of self-consciousness. Her emotions are fine.

I have characterized Delia's dream state. I have described its qualities and noted which of them are typical and which are significantly out of the ordinary. So now I will diagnose Delia's brain-mind state.

Delia has a typical case of dreaming. *That* seems quite certain: her brain-mind state is conscious and occurs in sleep; it is episodic; and it has consistent features. But what kind of psychosis does her dream represent? That is the question I wanted to answer, the question Jung and Freud never got to.

I have already pointed out that there is a clear dissimilarity between Delia's state and those with which dreaming has been commonly compared, namely schizophrenia and affective disorder. There is a clear similarity, however, between the main features of her dream state and those of an organic mental syndrome.

A syndrome is a collection of symptoms that crop up together in response to some pathological process. An organic brain syndrome is one that is caused by an anatomical or physiological alteration of the brain. People who are intoxicated with drugs or alcohol, have brain tumors, or have Alzheimer's disease have an organic mental syndrome. These three groups, by the way, often display parts of the following syndrome of features on the mental status exam:

1. Disorientation to time, place, and persons
2. Visual hallucinations
3. Distractibility and attention deficits

4. Recent memory loss
5. Loss of insight

These are the very characteristics of Delia's dream state that we found to be unusual! This leads us to the inescapable conclusion that dreaming *is* an organic mental syndrome!

Among the leading types of organic mental syndromes it is more like delirium than dementia. Delirium is commonly caused by sudden disruptions of brain functions, such as intoxication by impulsive overdosing of drugs, or a sudden stoppage in the use of drugs. As are other deliria, the visual hallucinations and the short-lived nature of the dream scenes suggest that the underlying cause of the dream state is a temporary instability or imbalance of physiology, rather than a permanent structural deficit.

What am I saying? Does Delia have a brain disease? Is she a closet junkie, an alcoholic? No. She is perfectly healthy and well adjusted. But her dream state matches the waking state of someone who has one of these problems. Unlike the anecdotal comparison of my own dreams with the psychotic episodes of Bertal, I have just performed a detailed clinical exercise to show that Delia's brain-mind dream state matches exactly the brain-mind waking state of someone who suffers from an organic mental syndrome.

Dreaming, then, is not *like* delirium. It *is* delirium. Dreaming is not a *model* of a psychosis. It *is* a psychosis. It's just a healthy one.

Now we begin to see how the brain-mind paradigm can pay off. We can study dreaming, we can manipulate it, and we can control it; it is a simple matter in a sleep lab. In doing so, we are studying, manipulating, and controlling a psychosis. If we can unveil the root cause of dreaming, we will have found the genesis of this psychosis.

Once we are powered with this knowledge, we can use it on the many other unhealthy psychoses that stalk people all around the globe. By understanding how the brain-mind produces a "normal" psychosis — dreaming — we may be able to understand how the brain-mind goes awry to produce a pathological psychosis. More broadly, if we can discern a set of principles and rules describing a normal conscious state and can alter that state experimentally, we

can deduce a set of principles and rules for altering abnormal conscious states — like Bertal's psychosis. Our ultimate goal is more
ambitious than solving the philosophical brain-mind problem; we
would like to solve the practical problems that damage the brain-
mind.

CHAPTER 4

The Cause of Delia's Delirium

[EVERY NIGHT in the emergency wards of hospitals in cities around the world ambulances bring in patients who are disoriented. Some are disheveled old bag ladies obsessed with the Last Judgment; some are rambling winos envisioning bugs climbing the walls; some are confused young men who just "woke up" in the city, having no idea how they got there or where they came from; and some are giddy young girls who don't even know their own names. Intrepid interns quickly assess the brain-mind states of these people by listing symptoms, in search of recognizable syndromes.

When a syndrome includes recent memory loss and confabulation, the doctors begin to construct menus of possible underlying organic diseases of the brain. Since these menus often get very long and the doctors don't want to miss anything easily treatable, they order basic lab tests: X-rays and CAT scans of the head, which could reveal major structural alterations of the brain caused by tumors or bleeding; electroencephalograms (EEGs), which could reveal functional alterations in the brain caused by epileptic seizures; and spinal fluid analyses, which could reveal infection or the ingestion of toxic chemical substances.

Since Delia's dream is a psychosis, similar tests performed while she is asleep could give us clues to the physiological cause of her nocturnal madness. And since Delia was so eager to learn more about her dreaming, I asked her if she would volunteer to undergo testing in my sleep lab. She said yes.

I told Delia I certainly didn't expect to observe structural problems in her head (which was a relief to her) and that my staff would therefore not take X-rays or CAT scans. But they would look for changes in brain electrical and chemical activity.

It would be an easy and painless matter to record the electrical activity of Delia's brain; my staff would hook her to an EEG machine while she slept. But how would they assess Delia's brain chemistry? Surely not by taking brain biopsies or withdrawing spinal fluid during her sleep. What they would do instead is apply what they already knew about brain chemistry as they observed her electrical activity and the body and eye movements she made while she slept. They had a good handle on brain chemistry thanks to scores of scientists who have studied extensively two of our fellow mammals — the cat and the rat — both of which have the same basic brain activity during sleep that humans do.

Animal models are used to study the biological underpinnings of all human brain dysfunctions. They have been crucial to the success that physicians have achieved so far in relieving the suffering associated with numerous neurological diseases. Polio, a nerve disease and the terror of my youth, is long gone because the virus that caused it and the vaccine that cured it were worked out on monkeys. The root causes of Parkinson's disease, which affects the same neurons in the brain stem that control the aminergic-cholinergic system, were found in rats. The pharmacology that led to the drug treatment now used was worked out on rats, too.

The same strategy is already proving essential in studying other brain-mind diseases, such as schizophrenia and Alzheimer's. In this regard, the basic science of the sleep research laboratory promises to play a key role in medical research.

As Delia slept, my staff and I would apply cellular and molecular evidence to explain the mechanisms of her psychosis. How would we know what to look for? To answer this crucial question we had to think a bit more critically and creatively about the syndrome we would try to explain.

REDUCING DELIA'S PSYCHOSIS

The great British neurologist John Hughlings Jackson, physician to the National Hospital for the Paralysed and Epileptic in London from 1862 to 1906, astutely observed that the loss of one brain-mind function in his patients was invariably associated with a reciprocal gain in another. Jackson linked this observation to Darwin's theory of evolution; as higher brain functions were added in evolution, lower functions were suppressed (but not lost). Jackson showed that when higher functions were lost in disease, lower functions reemerged to take their place.

In Delia's case, the mental status exam of her dream state indicated she had deficits in orientation, attention, memory, and insight; the reciprocal gains were in perception (the vivid hallucinations) and emotions (which were plentiful). The Hughlings Jackson within us might say that Delia's capacity to organize cognitive information (orientation, attention, memory, and insight) suffered at the expense of heightened sensations (perception and emotion).

Delia's four deficit functions had interlocking features, which suggested they might share some underlying brain mechanism. If so, the four cognitive losses could be reduced to one cause, a single cellular process. What could that process be? We didn't know, but intuitively we thought that what was missing was restraint, control, and stability. The basic restraining process of the brain is called inhibition.

To explain the enhanced sensations of Delia's psychosis — the hallucinations and emotions — we supposed that just as something had been subtracted from the system — restraint — something else had been added — ebullient enthusiasm. The brain-level process that reveals itself as enthusiasm is excitation.

If the loss of restraint is caused by a failure of inhibition, that same failure would allow an increase in excitation. Comparing the functional losses and gains in this way suggests the possibility that all six unusual factors in Delia's dream psychosis could be reduced to one, a single loss that would be a prime mover of a complex but interlocking set of processes. That is what we would look for as Delia slept in our lab.

A GROGGY NIGHT

Delia arrived about 10:00 P.M. the next evening, a bit weary from a long day. Though she had seen a sleep lab briefly in college, she looked around again with a new curiosity, since she would actually be sleeping here and we would be watching her. The lab consists of three rooms in a row, each opening off a common hallway. There is a bedroom at the far end, a recording room in the middle, and a second bedroom at the near end. From the recording room, my staff can observe a volunteer in either bedroom through one-way glass in windows in the walls.

Each bedroom is comfortably furnished with a double bed, a small bedside bureau, and an adjoining bathroom. I brought Delia, our only sleeper this evening, to Bedroom 1, where she met Sandy, one of my technicians. Sandy would be monitoring Delia throughout the night from the recording room.

Once Delia had gotten settled in bed, Sandy began to fix silver electrodes to her skin with a simple conductive paste and gauze pads. Sandy placed one electrode just to the side of each of Delia's eyelids, which would record eye movements, four on various points on her scalp, which would record brain activity, and two under her chin, which would record muscle signals. The eight electrodes plugged into jacks in the headboard, and wires ran from there to an EEG machine in the recording room (that way, should Delia need to use the bathroom during the night, she could simply pull the leads from the jacks and walk with them, like pulling the jack from a stereo while wearing headphones).

The EEG machine, or polygraph, would record the data on seven of its channels, plus an eighth channel for time; a pen for each data channel would quiver back and forth as a reel of paper continually rolled through the machine, producing a perpetual graph that looks somewhat similar to a strip chart from a seismograph that monitors earthquake activity.

Delia lay down to relax while Sandy went to the recording room to test the setup. "Move your eyes from side to side," said Sandy, talking into a microphone as she watched Delia through the glass. The two pens linked to the two electrodes next to Delia's eyes jumped. "Move your eyes left," Sandy said, and as Delia complied the two pens jumped apart. "Now right." The two pens converged.

While this was happening the four pens recording Delia's electrical brain activity were sketching away. Sandy told Delia to close her eyes and relax, but even after Delia had done so the four pens kept at it. Delia's head, just like B. F. Skinner's, was not a black box after all. While she lay quietly with her eyes closed, her relaxed state produced a powerful alpha rhythm on the EEG.

Sandy told Delia the instruments were working fine and that she could go to sleep. Being a devotee of meditation, Delia was practiced at inducing a state of relaxed waking. She often used the relaxation technique to release stress that built up during the day from the hustle and bustle of her life as a data analyst in the banking industry. To initiate the process, Delia sometimes said a mantra or just let her mind go blank. Entering this relaxation state would help Delia fall asleep in the lab, because as you can imagine, it is not easy to nod off with a bunch of wires glued to your head.

Another important relaxation trick that Delia had learned was to reduce the tension in her muscles. In the lab bedroom, she could actually hear the faint chatter of the recording pens when she clenched her teeth or stretched, because the two electrodes placed on her chin picked up the electrical signals that the muscles there generate during contraction. So if she was ever going to get to sleep under these conditions, she would have to keep her muscle channel quiet, and the best way to do that, she quickly learned, was to let the tension flow from her body.

When Sandy was prepping Delia a few minutes earlier, she had explained the awakening protocol for the night. "Do your best to sleep naturally," Sandy told her, "and when you hear your name called, wake up as promptly but peacefully as you can and give us a report of anything that was going on in your mind before you were awakened."

Despite being keyed up and a bit self-conscious, Delia had simply told herself, "Okay, I'm going to fall asleep and show these science types what a New Ager can dream up when sleeping under the ridiculous conditions of these experiments." After ten minutes, she was out.

Meanwhile, in the recording room, Ali, an undergraduate student in cognitive science who was serving an apprenticeship in the lab, had entered. Sandy explained the strategy of the experiment to him. She said that the four brain channels that generate the actual electroencephalogram (EEG) readings would tell them about the activation state of the upper brain, where the data processing involved in memory (amnesia), thinking (delusion), seeing (hallucination), and storytelling (confabulation) takes place. The two channels of the electrooculogram (EOG) would tell them about the timing, direction, and speed of eye movements. The channel showing the electromyogram (EMG) would record muscle signals that resulted from movement commands the brain would give the body; some of the muscles under the chin mediate the facial expressions that result from dream emotions, and others twitch during intensely imagined dream movements of the trunk and limbs. The eighth channel would be used to display time and to record such experimental events as awakenings.

FRANTIC PENS, A MILITARY INSTALLATION, AND ELECTRIC CURRENTS

Once Delia fell asleep her brain-mind was put on automatic pilot, first winding down quickly into a deep, utterly unconscious trough, then climbing up again to a peak of wild internal excitement. This cycle of falling and rising brain-mind activation would repeat itself through the night as Sandy and Ali watched in fascination.

All people have a sleep cycle, and people of the same general age have a similar one. For most teenagers and adults, the sleep cycle repeats every 90 to 100 minutes. If you sleep from six to eight hours, you will go through four or five cycles.

Within each cycle there are four possible types of sleep. Stage 1 is a light sleep, Stage 2 deeper, Stage 3 deeper still, and Stage 4 the deepest. Each cycle usually begins with a quick descent through Stage 1 into Stage 2, then 3 or 4, and ends after an ascent back up, followed by a stretch of Stage 1 sleep. Picture stepping down a short flight of stairs, stopping at the bottom, stepping back up, and stopping at the top.

The deepest sleep is in Stage 4. When we first fall asleep, we usually proceed rapidly through other stages to Stage 4. During this stage, brain activity is severely limited, heart rate and respiration and body temperature are at their lowest, and we do not dream. Stage 3 and Stage 2 have similar characteristics; they are just less extreme. Stage 1 is when we are most likely to dream. The brain is very active, and heart and respiration rates increase significantly. Our eyes also dart back and forth behind our closed eyelids as they track the images we "see" as we dream. These rapid eye movements (REMs) are the well-known signature of dreaming. Stage 1 sleep is therefore called REM sleep, while the other stages are grouped into non-REM sleep. As we end each 90-minute cycle in Stage 1 REM sleep, we dream, with a possible exception in the final cycle, when we often awake instead. If you pass through five 90-minute cycles in a night, you will have four or five dream episodes. Considering that, it's amazing how few we remember.

Sandy and Ali let Delia sleep through the first two cycles, readily recognizable on the EEG chart, because non-REM sleep is prevalent and dreams are scant and short. As Delia ascended her silent staircase in the third cycle of the night, however, she had a prolonged, intense REM period. "It's a classic," Sandy said as the third rise of activity neared its peak. The EEG pens jumped frantically across the strip chart, the eye and muscle pens followed in sync.

"Look at those eye movements!" Ali exclaimed. "Her brain must be buzzing."

"This is the kind of brain-wave pattern that occurs when people are startled or frightened," said Sandy, who had studied the outcome of many sleep lab nights. "And even though her muscle tone is completely suppressed now, there are spikes in the EMG, which indicate twitches in the face, arms, and legs. Let's wake her up and ask her what's going on in her head."

Sandy grabbed the microphone right in the middle of a flurry of rapid eye movements. "Delia! . . . Delia!" she called in a strong but calm tone. "Delia, please wake up. Wake up and tell us what you see." Delia was groggy, but since she had already been asleep for more than four hours she came around. "What?" she asked.

"Delia, it's Sandy. Tell us what you were dreaming." Although Delia appeared a bit lethargic and disoriented, she quickly regained her cognitive bearings. She closed her eyes as if to replay the dream and described what she experienced.

I was in a tall building in a military installation where people were working on weaponry. An electrical device was fired from an airplane at the building. Electric currents traveled down the metal frame of the building, with the effect that the external shell of the building became hardened so that people could not easily escape.

Another weapon was used against the people of the building, with the effect that images of people walking through the halls were created so that real people might fall in line behind them and be thwarted from trying to escape. I was in a group of people who were still trying to escape. One of them told me to follow the people in the halls, since they were primarily illusory.

We broke through a window and got out before it was too late. It was dusk out. We wondered how dangerous it was outside the building — we were afraid people might be waiting outside to pick us off as we came out.

We made our way to a house. A man I was with captured some weapons from the house. He threw a handgun through a window of the house to me. We escaped down a railroad track, and the man told me to shoot whoever came after us. I fumbled with the weapon, so the man exchanged the rifle he had for the handgun he had given me, since he thought it might improve my aim.

That was it. A typical sleep lab specimen in that Delia felt menaced by electrical technology! "Okay, Delia," Sandy said. "Thanks. You can go back to sleep." Delia had already sunk her head back into the pillow. The noisy chatter of the muscle and eye polygraph pens went mute the moment she went back to sleep. The EEG pens quieted down too, resuming the typical pattern of the next non-REM sleep trough.

Sandy and Ali took a quiet look at the readings on the strip chart from the last few minutes. The difference in activity that correlated with Delia's dream, her non-REM sleep, her waking, and her subsequent sleep was striking. The regular, uneventful EEG pattern of the non-REM sleep indicated a low level of brain-mind activation. The period was suddenly punctuated by the sharply defined and distinctive plot of the REM-dreaming stage. Delia's description of her dream correlated well with the EEG, eye, and muscle readings during her REM sleep. In her dream there were many people and objects, conversations, and changing scenes to track, both mentally and with her eyes. She experienced several strong emotions — frustration, resistance, fear — which correlated with facial motions and muscle contraction.

I told Sandy and Ali that the traits of Delia's dream also matched nicely those I had observed when doing the mental status exam on her earlier dream report that we had examined in the class. Delia's dream psychosis on this night in the lab had the same noticeable deficits in orientation (she finds the Al-Aqsa Mosque in Paris), attention (she cannot focus on any person or object — the images simply stream past her), memory (she can't recognize people although she knows she works with them), and insight (she doesn't realize she is dreaming). She also had the same reciprocal gains in perception (the vivid hallucinations) and emotions (which pervaded both scenes). Delia's description of her own REM sleep was full of evidence of the negative and positive aspects of her psychosis.

WHAT THE SLEEP LAB FINDINGS MEAN

Delia continued to sleep. She was entering the non-REM portion of her fourth sleep cycle. Sandy and Ali took a preliminary look at the data. They saw that during REM, Delia's brain-mind was involved in a very dynamic process. Her EEG was strongly activated during her dream, evidence of the rich and vivid mental activity in her dream report. The internal motor signals that were being generated and read out as rapid eye movements and muscle twitches on the polygraph matched the visuomotor intensity of Delia's dream experience. The absence of signals from Delia's chin muscles, however, indicated a suppression of overt motor activity, and indeed Delia's physical behavior was suppressed. She wasn't, in fact, standing up in bed as she tried to break the windows and flee the military installation. She was lying quite still because her muscles were paralyzed by the spinal inhibition of REM sleep. Had Sandy and Ali recorded heart rate and respiration they undoubtedly would have seen the rapid rise and fall of pulse and breathing during that scene which typify anxiety states.

In non-REM sleep, Delia's brain-mind was in a state of less intense activation. Sandy and Ali had awakened Delia twice during non-REM sleep and asked for a report. Delia's reports were short and confused; there were no vivid images, no Dali-like visions, no scurrying about, no elaborate and improbable buildings, and no flying. Just prior to the awakenings, her brain-wave (EEG) pattern was slow. There was no evidence of visuomotor stimulation on the polygraph either, no eye movements, no muscle twitches, and no suppression of motor output.

Having studied the outcome of thousands of sleep lab experiments at Harvard and other institutions, Sandy has come to the following conclusions: When there is EEG evidence of brain activation in sleep, the person sleeping experiences a vivid form of consciousness. When the brain activation is associated with eye movements, the person perceives images clearly. When most muscle activity is suppressed but small twitches of the face, fingers, head, and limbs appear, the person imagines himself to be running, flying, or swimming. When the heart beats rapidly and breathing rate increases sharply, the person experiences panic anxiety.

All these detailed correlations, I told Sandy and Ali, have led us to consider the possibility that dreams are simply the brain-mind's awareness of its own fully automatic, self-activated state. There is no dream spirit that invades the body during sleep and leaves it again come morning (as the Greeks supposed). There is no dream soul that descends an angelic ladder during sleep and climbs it again before dawn (as the medieval Christians hypothesized). But there is the wondrous brain-mind with all of its creative power, which renders a totally convincing and dramatically powerful conscious experience using only its own energy and information. Just flip the switch and watch the show.

I told them, too, however, that the sleep lab findings have told us too little about what is happening within the brain itself. We needed to uncover some physical changes within the brain that correlated with the cognitive deficits of disorientation, attention failure, and loss of insight, and the enhancements of perception and emotion. We had to uncover what was subtracted from the waking mix in Delia's brain that would account for the negative features of her psychosis, and we needed to know what was added that would account for the enhanced features.

A LOOK INSIDE THE DREAMING BRAIN

Seated in the recording room, Sandy, Ali, and I began to discuss what was happening at the molecular level in Delia's brain, as she peacefully slept the rest of the night away next door. Luckily for us, a colleague of mine, Roberto, was around conducting some experiments in the animal lab downstairs, and he joined us.

Roberto is one of the best brain marksmen in the world. He has more than a decade of experience in placing minute recording probes and drug-delivery devices deep into brain tissue. He always seems to hit his targets, no matter how deeply buried in the brain they lie and no matter how small they are. And the electrical recordings that result from his probings are impeccable.

As you might guess, Roberto does not place probes in the brains of people. Even though the brain has no nerves of its own to signal pain, and even though it is not likely that a probe would cause any damage, neither Roberto nor I believe we will meet someone soon who will be willing to have a probe inserted into his brain.

Enter one of our favorite household pets, the cat, to a suitable round of applause. The cat's sleep pattern is strikingly similar to our own. Cats' brain waves, eye movements, and muscle twitches clearly differentiate waking, non-REM, and REM sleep in a manner that is parallel to what people experience. The cat's sleep cycle also has a clocklike regularity, except that it is about thirty minutes long instead of ninety. The cat's brain has no sensory nerves of its own, either, and as pet lovers know, cats are brilliant at falling asleep and staying that way.

The probes Roberto inserts into the brains of sleeping cats are so thin they can eavesdrop on the signals of individual cells and record the conversation for many minutes or even hours. The electrical activity is sent directly to an oscilloscope, and it is an amazing sight. The trace on the oscilloscope jumps in staccato fashion, and the clicks of the signals coming through the scope's speakers chatter away like the sound of a high-speed telegraph.

Roberto's recording of individual cells would be key to our discussion, because his work and that of others has shown that with each signal, specific chemicals are liberated from the cells. If enough brain-stem cells of a particular chemical type increased — or decreased — their signaling in unison, the whole brain might undergo a major change in its chemical state. Such a major change in chemical state could help us explain why Delia's brain is switched from waking to dreaming, just as Bertal's brain is switched from sane to crazy. It was the brain stem, too, that we would focus on, because we already knew that the cells in the brain stem that emit the neurotransmitters norepinephrine and serotonin shut off during dreaming, while the brain-stem cells that signal with acetylcholine discharge wildly. We already had a strong suspicion about what was being subtracted and added to Delia's brain to create her dream delirium.

The brain stem lies at the base of the back of the head, just above the top of the neck, and extends inward. Deep in the center of the brain stem is a region called the pons. Cognitive functions in the cortex, the upper part of the brain, are turned on by a sustained activation process that arises in the pons. Some repetitive motor functions like walking and running also begin with signals sent from the pons down the spinal cord. With his probes, Roberto has found that the motor messages are actually blocked during REM — the motor output is turned off. Only the eyes are free to fly around in their sockets, he said, in part because these movements are so imperceptible they don't wake cats or people. Sleep, it seems, is protected from disruption by motor inhibition.

The EEG waves that arise in the pons are called PGO waves, because they radiate from the pons (P) to the geniculate (visual) body (G) and the occipital (visual) cortex (O). During dreams, the shape of these waves resembles that of waves recorded during epileptic seizures. By understanding how the brain normally produces and controls this seizure-like activity, some brain researchers hope to learn new ways to reduce the suffering of people with epilepsy.

Research into epilepsy, Roberto told Sandy and Ali, offered us another clue. The temporal lobes (hidden behind the temples next to our ears) are one part of the brain that is particularly prone to seizures. They are also the seat of emotion. If there was a way to figure out how the PGO waves are turned on in REM — and turned off in the other brain-mind states — we would not only have a strong clue as to the cause of the visuomotor hallucinations, but also a leg up on how the emotional brain gets into seizure-like states that cause the wild anxiety of some of our dreams and the dreamlike states of some psychotic patients.

Roberto was leading them on, I knew, because he and colleagues had already conducted experiments on cats that would furnish an answer. They had selected a synthetic molecule called carbachol, which resembles acetylcholine. They then injected it into the pons of cats that were awake or in non-REM sleep, and the cats suddenly switched to REM sleep and (we might suppose) began to dream. The carbachol set the REM process in motion throughout the rest of the brain.

Since carbachol mimics the action of acetylcholine, they concluded, it is acetylcholine that triggers the PGO waves. These waves, in turn, initiate the visual hallucinations and emotions of dreams. Although the proof was indirect, it was compelling; a buildup of acetylcholine, which would develop progressively in Delia's brain stem during non-REM sleep, would initiate REM sleep. The whole dream experience might thus be triggered by a single molecule.

Could this really be? Sandy and Ali wondered. Roberto recounted the experimental evidence brain scientists had found in recent years that supported the idea. First, he noted, the pons is a crucial part of the visual system; the cells that execute all our eye movements are located there. So are the cells that turn muscle tone on and off and program our gaits like walking and running, and acetylcholine is involved in mediating some of these actions; in fact, researchers can turn walking or running on and off by stimulating the pons. The PGO system also tells the sensory part of the visual brain what the motor part is doing, and it uses acetylcholine to relay that information. What the visual brain does with the acetylcholine signals during REM sleep is hallucinate; that's what we think happens to the cats when carbachol is squirted into their pons.

A CHEMICAL BALANCING ACT

The step that remained was to figure out what turned on the acetylcholine system in the pons in the first place. Could it be that the acetylcholine network was always ready to take over but was held in restraint by inhibitory signals from some other network? The answer is a resounding yes.

It is only recently that scientists were stunned to discover how much is actually going on inside the brain during sleep. Once scientists had gotten used to their counterintuitive discovery that internal brain functions persist at high levels in sleep, they gave up the idea that the brain itself ever really rests. Then some cells were discovered in the pons whose activity decreased to about half during non-REM sleep and was virtually arrested during REM sleep while the rest of the brain was active at near seizure levels. What did the cells contain? Norepinephrine and serotonin — the amines.

The amines' role in the pons is to decide what to do with messages that are generated within the cells there. They decide to respond or not respond, to record or not record, to store or not store. When we are awake, these cells fire and secrete amines continuously, which among other things restrains the cholinergic system. The biggest clusters of serotonin cells lie right down the middle of the pons, and the norepinephrine cells lie on either side of them.

From these sites they all project great distances all the way up to the cortex and down to the spinal cord. This reach is much more widespread than that of the acetylcholine system.

Once Delia began to relax in Bedroom 1 way back around 10:30 or so, the neurons in her pons that contain amines quieted down enough for her to enter non-REM sleep. The cells fired more and more slowly. Fewer and fewer of the amines were secreted into her brain. The electrical drive on her cortex fell. The relative strength of the acetylcholine system, though still in abeyance during non-REM sleep, was building.

After 70 or 80 minutes something funny happened. The system switched. Activity in the cells containing the amines, which had been drifting amiably downward, plunged to its lowest level of the day; the secretion of amines plunged with it. As the nose-dive ensued, the activity of neighboring cells containing acetylcholine soared to a peak rarely experienced even under intense stimulation during waking. Acetylcholine was secreted in abundance. Delia's brain had changed its chemical mind.

No one yet knows exactly how the amine neurons are silenced, but the lack of restraint on Delia's cholinergic system by norepinephrine and serotonin was nearly total. Delia's brain-mind came under the complete domination of the cholinergic system. Fueled by acetylcholine, her visuomotor circuits buzzed away. It was anything goes in the image, idea, and feeling factory. Her brain-mind was like a pinball machine with all its lights flashing.

When Delia entered REM sleep and began to dream, the motor-pattern generators of her brain stem and upper brain were turned on. Motor commands like "run" or "break the windows" were emitted and Delia felt as if she were really running or trying to get away in a hurry. Fortunately for Delia, however, those same commands were not relayed to her muscles because her spinal motor nerves were paralyzed by inhibition.

Delia's brain-mind called up scenes to fit the emotion of fear. The scenes were peopled with dramatis personae from her fear fantasy file. Because of the lack of restraint on her cortex, Delia's capacity to confabulate was enhanced. Anonymous characters with guns would do for the story. This loosening of associations was not entirely without rhyme or reason, however; there was an underlying set of rules constraining the scenario structure of the dream, because it did make a lot of sense given the fact that she was wired up to an EEG machine!

Given all that has been said so far, it is not hard to see why Delia's attention failed in her dream psychosis. There was no way for her to focus on one of the multiple competing streams of internally generated imagery arising in response to her overactive brain stem. First one percept gained center stage, then another, in chaotic fashion.

When she was dreaming, Delia's brain-mind also switched from top-down control, where volition has an important say in what happens, to bottom-up control, where volition is swept away. Therefore her loss of control over thought is understandable. Thinking is like a motor act in that it requires top-down control. But those PGO waves rolling over her brain and those showers of acetylcholine dampen any spark that persists of the "I" that watches, weighs, and wills her actions when she is awake. In REM sleep Delia is still sure of her own identity, but she is not at all in command of her acts. Things just happen to her and she tries, in vain, to figure them out. This dissolution of will in dreams has always posed a severe threat to many ethicists, who are disturbed to think that such a precious human trait as conscience is so fragile as to be dissolved by a change in state.

The scientific evidence now seems clearly in favor of an even more radical conclusion. Not only is volition dependent upon the state of the brain-mind, volition *is* a state of the brain-mind. The good news is that, to a degree, we can make up our minds. The bad news is that, to a degree, we cannot. It is our sometimes psychotic minds that make *us* up.

Why did Delia's dream end? Because the flood of acetylcholine was turned off immediately when her serotonin and norepinephrine neurons turned back on. As the two amines flowed back toward her cortex, Delia's capacity to focus, recall, and remember came back too. Why Delia is so good at remembering the content of her dream state, when others are so bad, however, is still a complete mystery.

By now it was nearly 6:00 A.M. and Delia began to wake up. Sandy, Ali, Roberto, and I, however, were ready for some sleep of our own. Sandy removed the electrodes from Delia, and we all invited her to visit our scientific hotel again. She went off for a shower and breakfast. We went off for our beds — at home.

LEARNING FROM PSYCHOSIS

Now we finally have a complete answer to the two key questions posed earlier about Delia: What kind of psychosis is her dreaming? And what causes it? The mental status exam showed us that Delia's dream psychosis is a delirium. The sleep lab experiment informed us that it is caused by a shift in the chemical balance within her brain. There is indeed, as I had hypothesized along with Hughlings Jackson at the outset of this chapter, a single process that caused the six cognitive losses and gains of Delia's delirium; it is the loss of aminergic inhibition and the reciprocal gain in cholinergic excitation.

The most important implication of these conclusions is that alterations of the conscious states of the brain-mind obey reliable and specifiable rules. Whether the states are a normal delirium, like dreaming, or an abnormal delirium, like alcohol withdrawal, they always have the same formal features and the same kind of cause. The common features of normal and abnormal delirium are disorientation, inattention, impoverished memory, confabulation, visual hallucinations, and abundant emotions. The common cause of normal and abnormal delirium is a sudden shift in the balance of brain chemicals. If norepinephrine, serotonin, or acetylcholine levels change suddenly, all hell breaks loose.

Knowing the shared features of all kinds of delirium and their common underlying cause is a huge payoff from the brain-mind paradigm. The paradigm unites a set of normal and universal phenomena, those seen in dreaming, with a pathological and exceptional set of phenomena, those seen in organic psychosis. This tour de force not only builds the piers of the brain-mind bridge but it allows normal and abnormal conscious states to march across it hand in hand. The promised land that can be reached by crossing the brain-mind bridge is a space in which all the myriad variations of our conscious experience could be defined and explained.

In chapter 5, we will explore that space.

Traveling in Brain-Mind Space

I N THE 1960s when Mercury capsules and Sputniks were hurling humans into earth orbit, the hip culture experimented with what came to be called head trips. Instead of rocket fuel, these psychedelic voyages into inner space were propelled by drugs like LSD and mescaline, which alter brain-mind states chemically. We now know that street drugs such as acid and angel dust cause hallucinations because they are chemically similar to the natural molecules that initiate dreaming, and they interact with the neurons that control the states of waking and REM sleep.

It is no accident that the drug-induced visions of psychedelic fame are so dreamlike. Nor can we resist describing our dreams as psychedelic. Prompted by these compelling analogies we want to create a unified framework for thinking about our inner space. How do we travel from waking to sleep to dreaming during the course of each day and night? What holds us on a normal course? And what causes some of us to go off track into the forbidden zones of delirium, psychosis, or coma?

In this chapter I'll develop a three-dimensional model of brain-mind space to answer these questions. Then I'll use the model to integrate what I have learned about Delia's dream psychosis with Bertal's waking psychosis. The result will be the outline of a model of all brain-mind states.

WHAT MADE DELIA DREAM?

A list of all the possible conscious and unconscious states would be quite lengthy. Let's consider what the key factors are that drive all the brain-mind states. If there is only one, then a linear model, like the spectrum of colors of visible light, might do; if there are two, then a two-dimensional graph will do; if there are three, then a three-dimensional model, like a sphere or cube, is needed.

When Sandy and Ali had finished recording Delia's sleep on that long night in the sleep lab, they trudged wearily downstairs carrying a box of folded chart paper weighing about ten pounds and extending — when laid out end to end — about a thousand feet. Eight pens had continuously traced various aspects of Delia's brain-mind state over the seven and a half hours she was in the lab: her brain waves, her muscle tone, her eye movements. There were seven thousand feet of data — a mile and a third of it — to analyze.

Once Sandy and Ali had themselves slept and were again alert enough to think straight, they began to score Delia's record, page by page. They retraced Delia's night life to see what the fundamental factors were that correlated with her periods of non-REM sleep, REM sleep, and waking.

One fundamental factor was the electrical activity within Delia's brain. As the electrical power in her brain declined, her consciousness faded, just like the light of a chandelier when someone slowly turns down a dimmer switch. When the electrical power was turned back up, the lights came on, and Delia was in REM sleep. One key factor, then, is electrical activation.

But why doesn't Delia wake up to the outside world when the power comes back on? And why can't she control the thoughts, feelings, and memories of her dreams in REM? Because as the brain is internally reactivated in REM, sensory input from the outside world is actively blocked; her brain can't receive and process external data. Her motor output also is held in check, so she can't act out her dreams; she didn't actually move her legs as she fled the military installation and she didn't actually move her arms as she caught the handgun that was tossed to her.

However, by analyzing the long strip chart, Sandy and Ali saw that Delia's eyes moved back and forth as she envisioned the aspects of her dreams. So her brain-mind was indeed seeing the objects of her dreams, as her eyes moved automatically. What happened was that Delia switched from an external source of visual data to an internally generated source. She changed from external inputs to internal inputs. A second key factor, then, is the input source.

There was still a problem; the changes in electrical activation and the input source could not account for why Delia was not able to think straight during her dreams, why she didn't realize she was dreaming when she was dreaming, and why she couldn't remember all her dreams. Apparently, her mode of information processing had changed when she dreamed. It changed from rational, logical, and self-aware (the traits of being awake), to delusional, illogical, and unreflective (the traits of dreaming). The third critical factor, then, is mode. The mode of the brain-mind depends on the aminergic-cholinergic control system — on whether the amines are in power, the cholines are in power, or the two are deadlocked.

Sandy and Ali found that these three factors — activation energy, input source, and mode of processing — could account for all the experiences Delia had during her night in the lab and for all the variants in the readings they analyzed on the strip chart. A brief look at the clock once they had finished this exercise, however, reminded them there was a fourth factor: time. The degree to which the three key factors are in effect changes continually over time.

Now that we recognize that there are three factors that mediate the various states we experience during sleep and that these vary over time, we can create a model that describes our brain-mind space. This model is the essence of the brain-mind paradigm.

THE THREE DIMENSIONS
OF BRAIN-MIND SPACE

Let's call the key factors for our model A for activation energy, I for information source, and M for mode. Let's put time on the back burner for the moment. The labels of the three dimensions read AIM, a fortuitous acronym.

Since there are three factors, we can pick any three-dimensional shape we want for our model. The simplest is a cube — a die to play Monopoly, a Rubix Cube game, a racquetball court, an empty box.

Since we're making all this up, we can put the three dimensions along any of the edges of the cube. Imagine holding a box in front of you at eye level; let A represent the width, I the depth, and M the height of the box. If you were in a school auditorium looking head-on at the stage, A would run from left to right, I from front to rear, M from the floor to the ceiling.

It is important to recognize that the state-space model we have just constructed is entirely artificial. Like other scientific models, it is a model, built to help us represent and test a theory. It also will help us visualize how the brain-mind changes state.

Let's check that the model makes sense. Is it realistic? Yes; the dimensions and values are drawn from specific data taken in the sleep lab. Is it dynamic? Yes; it recognizes the continuously shifting nature of brain-mind states. Is it comprehensive? Yes; the space has an infinite number of points or positions within it, so all possible states of the system can be accommodated. Is it continuous? Yes; there are no qualitative boundaries separating the normal from the abnormal in the three-dimensional space. Is it predictive? Yes; if we change one factor, we can see how that will affect the other two.

Let's visualize how this model can represent a few of the basic brain-mind states. Take a seat in the auditorium and look at the empty stage.

Now imagine a dot hovering in the cubic space. Place it, say, in the right, back, upper corner of the space. Color it red just to liven things up a bit. As long as the dot hovers more or less in this sector it represents a stable state, because its position — representing the three properties of activation, information source, and mode of processing — doesn't change very much.

Which state is the dot in? The left-to-right axis is activation; activation is low to the left, high to the right. So the activation energy is high. The front-to-back axis is information source; front is the internal source, back is the external. So the information source is external. The floor-to-ceiling axis is mode; when acetylcholine is in power, the mode is at the floor; and when the amines are in power, the mode is at the ceiling (when the two are deadlocked, the mode is halfway up). So the mode is aminergic. Thus, when the dot is in the right, back, upper corner, the brain-mind state is highly activated, information is coming from the outside world, and the amines are clicking away. We are awake!

Getting tired of this? So tired you want a nap? Then move the dot. As you get sleepy the activation of your brain decreases; the dot moves from the right side of the stage toward the left. You close your eyes, decreasing the external inputs; the dot moves from the rear of the stage forward. You doze off, losing rational thought as acetylcholine battles to retake control from the amines; the dot moves from the ceiling of the stage down toward the floor. The dot is now in the center of the cube; you are in non-REM sleep.

Where would the dot be if you were to really zonk out for a while and begin to dream? On the floor, in the front, right-hand corner. During dreaming, acetylcholine is in control, so your mode would be all the way down on the floor. The inputs are fully internal, which correlates with the very front of the stage. But recall that brain activity increases greatly during REM; the activation energy is high again, placing the dot all the way to the right, as it was during waking.

We can move the dot to any region of the cube and imagine the consequences. Where would Bertal's dot be when he was running from the dive-bombers? In the right, top, *front* corner, as opposed to the right, top, *back* corner that is normal waking. Bertal's activation is high (the right), the amines are in power (top), but his processing mode has switched its attention from the normal external inputs (back) given by his eyes and ears to an abnormal internal source (front) that is generating hallucinations.

Where does the dot lie for a hospital patient in coma? At the left, bottom, front corner. It is at the left because there is virtually no brain activation, at the bottom because acetylcholine is in domination, and at the front because there is no recognition of external sensations, meaning the brain is processing only internal information. A mother and father will sit endlessly at the bedside of their daughter who has lapsed into coma following a tragic accident and talk to her and rub her hands in a desperate attempt to "get through" to her. In rare cases the child's eyes may flicker or her hand may twitch; the parent's well-known voice or touch is an external source of information that may activate the brain, for only an instant, in a vain attempt to jolt the dot of the comatose child from its depth at the front left corner of the stage floor. As anyone who has witnessed prolonged coma knows, the brain-mind of the poor child has become stuck in the corner and will never get out. And should the activation value go to zero, it's all over. Brain death has occurred.

FINE-TUNING THE AIM MODEL

Now that we have a basic understanding of the AIM model, let's look at the three dimensions more closely, to see how they contribute to moving us from one brain-mind state to another.

Activation (A)

The activation function represents the amount of electrical activity going on in the brain. It can be estimated from the frequency of an EEG. It is also a measure of the rate at which most neurons are firing in the brain.

The concept of activation has strong roots in the brain-mind sciences. In neurology, it accounts for the switching on of the upper brain in both waking and REM sleep. In psychology, it is used to interpret results of memory studies; in order to remember something, we have to activate a set of connected cells that encode the data.

The idea of activation also has become the central concept of neural networks, the software that runs the so-called artificial intelligence computers. Whether or not neural networks can learn by changing their properties over time, the probability of getting *any* output from an input into a computer, or our brains, is a function of the level of activation (or "drive" or "power"). No activation, no processing. Lots of activation, lots of processing.

Again, low values of activation are to the left in the AIM cube, high values to the right. As we raise the level of activation the dot moves from left to right, no matter how high, low, deep, or shallow it is in the brain-mind space. We can run the dot from side to side at will, thus activating or deactivating the system.

Information Source (I)

This factor tells us whether the data we are processing comes mainly from the outside world (as it does when we are awake and attentive) or from inside our heads (as it does when we lapse into fantasy or when we dream).

There is considerable evidence from both experimental psychology and neurology that perception is a collaboration between representations brought to our brains by our senses and information already encoded there in memory. Consider how we identify an image. When I come out of my office and head for my conference room, I often see the coat rack in the hallway. In the summer, when there are no coats or hats on it, it is just a coat rack. But let the weather change and I begin to have trouble seeing it only for what it is. In winter, when there is both a coat and a hat on the rack, I often catch the image out of the corner of my eye and am startled, because I think for an instant it is a person standing there. My head and eyes are drawn to this imaginary person frequently, even though I know better.

You probably have had similar experiences, especially in the dark, when you are alone and anticipating danger. Everything that rustles, glitters, or moves is — until proven otherwise — an attacker. You have to talk to yourself so as to not overreact. In psychology, this is called projection, and it always occurs when the balance of input strength shifts from external to internal.

There is a constant interplay between information coming in from the external world and our internally stored images. As long as our expectancies and observations match, we are comfortable. But let the internal imagery (our imagination) become too strong and we either misperceive the outside world, or become anxious, or both. Here we recognize that emotion and perception are in constant interaction. Misperceptions increase our anxiety, and anxiety increases our misperceptions. This vicious cycle can lead to neurosis and even to psychosis.

During waking the relative strength of external to internal stimulation is high and, as with the coat rack, is subject to immediate correction via focused attention. But funny things begin to happen as the strength of the external stimuli diminish, either due to darkness or because our brains are not so highly activated when we are getting sleepy. It is in the dark and at the edges of sleep that microhallucinations most commonly arise.

Thus the AIM variable I, the information or input source, exists along a continuum, just like the level of activation. In the AIM cube, the information level runs from purely internal, at the front of the stage, to purely external, at the back of the stage.

Note, now, that when the dot is at the right front of the stage, it has high activation and strong internal input, regardless of whether it is near the ceiling or the floor. This is the column of hallucination, if you will. When Delia is dreaming, her dot is at the right front, on the floor; her brain activation is high, and the visual information is generated internally, but the cholinergic system has control, keeping her asleep. When Bertal sees dive-bombers, he too is at the right front, but is up at the ceiling; his brain activation is high, and the visual information is generated internally, but the aminergic system has control, meaning that he is awake. And since the column has a midsection it allows us to account for random images that sometimes arise in non-REM sleep.

Mode (M)

Whether the aminergic or cholinergic system is in power is described as the mode of the brain-mind state. The aminergic-cholinergic system modulates cognition — attention, volition, insight, and so on, all of which differ so radically between waking and dreaming.

It is the M function that enables the activated brain-mind to select, hold, and evaluate its representations when we are awake. We call this thinking or analytic reasoning. In dreaming, we can't think in this way. Recall that both the aminergic and cholinergic systems are always active; M is the ratio of the relative power of amines to cholines. A high value of M represents the relative dominance of amines when we are awake. A low value of M means that the amines are repressed and acetylcholine is dominant. We are dreaming. We have no volition (we can't stop the dream). We have no control over our attention (we can't take a closer look at a passing flower or a pizza shop). Moreover, a great paradox ensues when we wake up: although our memories are released during dreams, we usually cannot remember the dream.

As is the case with the other two variables, the ratio of amines to acetylcholine exists along a continuum. In the AIM model, the highest value of the ratio is at the ceiling, the lowest value is at the floor.

Brain research shows that there is a direct link between cell metabolism and the aminergic-cholinergic ratio. Recall that the two amine neuromodulators are norepinephrine and serotonin. They may inhibit or excite the neurons. But they also redirect the metabolic activity of the neuron cells they contact. Thus when a cell is contacted, say, by norepinephrine, its firing may be inhibited, but it also may simultaneously be instructed to increase or decrease its metabolic activity, for example, or to synthesize a certain protein. Once this is done, the nature of the cell has changed. This is one proposed mechanism for the way in which brain cells "store" memories. The same activity may be responsible for learning, for locking in trauma, or for liberating a psychosis.

Because it can affect cell metabolism, this power of the aminergic-cholinergic system to control the mode of the brain is also crucial to the fundamental bodily phenomenon we call our health. This is because the aminergic and cholinergic systems of the brain stem have direct connections downward to the body. I will explore this further in later chapters.

MOVING IN AIM SPACE

I have spent considerable time describing the AIM model because it can be used to explain how we humans move from one brain-mind state to another. It can explain how we fall asleep, how in our sleep we alternate between non-REM and REM sleep, and how we wake up again the next morning. It also gives us strong clues as to what goes awry when people like Bertal "go crazy."

Let's visualize once again the dot, which represents the brain-mind state. Since you are now awake, your dot is hovering in the upper, back, right-hand corner of the cube, the domain of normal waking. Your activation level is high, you are processing external inputs, and the strength of your aminergic modulating system is high.

If your dot wanders away from the corner along any of the three axes, however, you will drift away from waking. One point is clear: normal waking is statistically improbable! If it were left to chance, you would be in this part of the cube only a small fraction of the time, yet you are "there" more like two-thirds of the time.

If you move your awake dot from the upper, back, right-hand corner toward the very middle of the cube, you are simulating the process of falling asleep. As the activation level falls, the ability of external data to control your thoughts also falls, and the power of the aminergic system weakens. When you are firmly in the center of the cube, you are in deep non-REM sleep. All systems are at half-throttle, and none overpowers the other. However, you remain in this stable state for only a while. Acetylcholine, having weakened the power of the amines, starts to take over, dragging your dot toward the floor. Your capacity to process external data falls precipitously; as it weakens, the internal data in your cognitive unconscious becomes powerful enough to create imagery (hallucination) and narrative (confabulation). And the acetylcholine reactivates your brain. Your dot, already sinking to the floor, is therefore pulled forward by the relative strength of internal information and to the right by the increasing activation. It stops in the bottom, front, right-hand corner of the cube. You are in dreamland.

How do you wake up? The amines never give up. There is a

buildup of tension between the amines and the acetylcholine; remember, their control is relative. At some point the tension snaps, and the amines leap back to power, which also changes your focus to external information. You have jumped to the upper, back, right-hand corner of the AIM cube.

Let's test this explanation for waking in another way. Suppose you are dreaming, and your good friend sneaks up to you and claps his hands loudly right next to your ears. You jump to attention (and proceed to throttle him for his kindness). But what happens in the AIM model? The external input is so strong it interrupts the internal input; it thrusts you from the front to the back of the stage. This shock alerts the amines (like any animal, we suddenly "power up" when we are shocked or threatened); they leap to power and thrust you from the floor to the ceiling. You are awake. Wide awake.

In this way we can explain the pharmacology of our everyday lives. For many of us, it's hard to "get up" once we wake up, especially if we have awakened to an alarm clock instead of our natural rhythms. And what do many of us look for to help us get it together? A cup of coffee. Coffee contains caffeine, a chemical stimulant. Caffeine affects us in the same way that amines do; it raises the activation level of our brains. By drinking coffee in the morning, we are trying to aid our bodies in shifting from one brain-mind state to another. Note, too, that when we drink coffee at night we are artificially trying to prevent our bodies from shifting back from the awake state to the sleeping state, again by raising our activation level and staving off the rising tide of acetylcholine.

What happens when we are suddenly threatened? We focus intently. Our senses peak. We ready our bodies for fight or flight. We are in a state of superactivation. Why? The adrenal gland releases adrenaline, a hormone; adrenaline is an aminergic molecule, and it heightens our activation as it simultaneously raises blood sugar and stimulates the heart. At the same time, aminergic molecules are released throughout the brain, and the neural circuits that control attention, anxiety analysis, and decision making are revved up to peak levels.

In animal sleep labs, researchers can cause cats that are awake to suddenly dream by giving them a small shot of carbachol, a chemical similar to acetylcholine; it shifts the mode to the cholinergic floor and moves the cats quickly into REM sleep. Obviously, we can't shoot carbachol into the human brain. But we can inject similar compounds into the veins of sleeping people; when we do, they slip more rapidly into REM sleep, stay there longer, have many more eye movements, and dream intensely.

And what happened to my friend Bertal? When he beat up my supervisor, we injected him with chlorpromazine. Suddenly he was calm and would sit to actually talk about his mother. His hallucinations stopped. When Bertal saw the dive-bombers, two of his three AIM factors were fine; his amines were in control (he was awake), and his activation was high (he could yell and run). But the part of his brain that processes visual imagery switched from monitoring the normal external inputs to the abnormal internal inputs. We now know that chlorpromazine affects another modulatory chemical — dopamine (an amine) — that we haven't yet been able to incorporate into our AIM model, but which we know interacts with the other amine and choline modulators. Once Bertal had the help of this drug, his input function was shifted from internal to external and he returned to normal waking.

We must tie up one loose end: time. Time was the fourth factor critical to our brain-mind states. The three AIM factors all change continuously over time. Time is represented simply by the movement of our dot; as time marches on, our dot moves back and forth between brain-mind states in the AIM model.

When we look at our daily trajectory through the state space, we cannot help but be impressed with the reliability of the restricted path that we normally follow. It resembles the shape of a boomerang, with one tip in the upper, back, right-hand corner (waking), the midsection in the center of the cube (non-REM sleep), and the other tip in the lower, front, right-hand corner (REM). That we do not normally enter most sectors of the cube is another way of saying that the system is self-limiting. For this we can be grateful in two ways. First, most of us are spared the indignities that beset patients like Bertal. And second, we have a better chance of understanding and influencing our movement through the state space because it occurs along a somewhat narrow and well-bounded corridor.

CURING PSYCHOSES

Using the AIM model, we now have a way to understand how the three key factors control all brain-mind states. These three forces — activation energy, information source, and modulation — dictate the state we are in at every moment in our lives. They are simple, but powerful.

Knowing this, we finally have a way to define in detail the many brain-mind states. Reaching this capability has been the goal of the first part of this book. The brain and the mind are not separate entities linked in some well-tuned way. They are one entity. That entity exists in various states. The states are controlled by three key variables, and as they vary, our brain-minds move from one state to another.

You can use the AIM model to think about your own brain-mind states. In presenting the model, I am not attempting to take away the wonderful, cozy feeling you may have about your dreams; they are no less magical just because you understand how they are created. I am not attempting, either, to challenge your beliefs about eternal life; I am attempting to describe with scientific rigor how the brain-mind works while you are on this earth, regardless of whether you think you are reincarnated or have a soul that will carry on after you are dead.

The minor discomforts of the brain-mind that we experience, from fatigue to anxiety to occasional sleeplessness, occur when one of the three key drivers is off a bit for some reason. Major mental illnesses such as schizophrenia and Alzheimer's, however, occur when there is a problem with one or more of the major faculties we possess, regardless of whether the cause is physical or psychological. These faculties are orientation, memory, perception, emotion, attention, and energy. In Part Two, I will examine each faculty and show how it is affected by the brain-mind states, and thus how the states can be used to correct the mental illnesses.

If we can figure out how each faculty works in a healthy state, we have a good chance of figuring how to fix it in an unhealthy state. The brain-mind state we best understand today is dreaming. Dreaming is not like a psychosis, it is a psychosis. It's just a healthy one. If we can monitor and experiment on the faculties during the healthy dream psychoses of people like Delia, we can then find the cause and perhaps treat the faculty problems that cause the unhealthy psychoses of people like Bertal.

PART TWO

ANALYZING THE BRAIN-MIND

CHAPTER 6

Lost and Found: Orientation and Disorientation

Y BEDROOM in Boston faces south, as does my bed, which hugs the north wall of the room. There are windows to the east, which are on my left as I sleep, and to the south, beyond the foot of the bed. Beyond the door in the wall to my right (the west) is that important antechamber to the great hall of sleep, the bathroom.

One recent morning I was awakened by a faint but definite clinking sound in the bathroom. Two years ago, before my daughter left for college, I would have slept right through this gentle noise, because her bedroom has a door to the bathroom from the other side. But I knew there should be no such sound to my right now, and I responded with alarm. My daughter was gone and there was no guest using her room.

How quickly this computation was made I can't accurately say, but I would guess it took all of about two seconds. My orientation process was as follows: (1) The place is my bedroom; there is no doubt about that because I am me, waking up in bed. (2) It's early morning because I can see a faint light through the drapes covering the east window and I am already aware of having gotten up during the night to use the bathroom.

Now that my brain-mind was more fully activated, I wondered who could possibly be making the sound in the bathroom. My orientational search for a candidate was powerfully driven by anxiety, an emotion that had been immediately activated by my not knowing *who*.

In that instant of waking, I went through a likely persons checklist. Was the *who*: (1) My daughter? No, she was away at college. (2) My live-in housekeeper? No, she never used that bathroom because there is another one immediately adjacent to her own quarters in the back of the house. (3) An overnight guest? No, I knew there was none. (4) My father? Impossible, his apartment is even more remote than my housekeeper's and at age ninety he doesn't wander.

Since I had eliminated all the innocent suspects, my anxiety rose another notch and I moved into the domain of menace. Had someone come in off the street? Unlikely, since I had locked the ground-floor doors and windows before retiring, as I do every night. Still, we had had two break-ins and one was by a second-story specialist. So it could be a crook. I imagined it was a man, because housebreakers are usually men, and because there had been a recent upsurge in neighborhood violence. I was by this time a plus-five on the five-point anxiety scale.

Although I was awake, I was as disoriented as I am in a dream. Except that my critical logic was working quite well; in a dream I don't reject the candidates that I call up to play a role. They simply pass by me. I even asked myself, Now why would any housebreaker be in my bathroom? There's nothing to steal in a bathroom.

The lights were coming up a bit, but not enough to protect me from a wild projection when I heard a faintly audible female voice in the bathroom. It must be the housebreaker's girlfriend and she's brushing her teeth, I thought.

Seriously! A professor at the Harvard Medical School came up with this nutty conclusion. But imaginative though I may sometimes be, I couldn't buy it. So I figured, I must be wrong about my whereabouts; I'm lost in the map room of my mind. My self-reflective awareness was telling me that I was barking up the wrong tree and that there was something wrong with my basic assumptions about space. I realized, still dimly, that I might be disoriented.

My anxiety level dropped to three and I began to regroup. Wait a second, I thought, my bedroom is almost never this dark and there should be light through the south windows, too. And then I heard *two* female voices. No housebreaker would take two girlfriends on the same job, I deduced, clinching the case: I must be in some other bedroom.

Sure enough, I *was* in another bedroom. I had just awakened in a hotel in Columbus, Ohio. Out in the hallway, just beyond the bathroom, were two chambermaids clearing the room opposite of a room-service tray and clinking the glasses on it. It is important to note that the bath of the hotel room *was* on my right as I lay in that bed, which did hug the bedroom's north wall; I was lying in the same relative position with respect to the east window of the hotel, through which the sunrise light really did filter as I woke up. In my terror, however, I was roughly six hundred miles to the west of my Boston bedroom.

There are several points to this story. The first is that our sense of orientation is a construction that we have to fabricate upon awakening every day. The second is that if we have even one important detail wrong, orientation is difficult or even impossible. The third is that other aspects of our consciousness, such as our ability to think straight and to feel calm, are dependent upon our being oriented. The fourth is that our ability to orient is strongly state dependent; if five minutes rather than five seconds had elapsed between my awakening and my hearing a noise, I would have had no trouble knowing what was going on. Finally, this vignette illustrates that there is a tight link between thinking and feeling; and there is a very strong and decidedly counterproductive feedback loop between anxiety and disorientation. The more anxious I became, the more outlandish were the ideas I entertained to explain the noises in what I mistakenly took to be my Boston bathroom.

My small case of mental illness quickly corrected itself. Indeed, so quickly did I get my bearings that I would never have taken any notice of the episode — my mind jumped through all those hoops in what was probably less than two minutes — had I not primed myself during the preceding months to try to pay attention to the process of waking up. How, I wondered, could a system so badly out of whack in one state (dreaming) right itself so quickly and so thoroughly in a new state (waking)?

This story also illustrates that brain-mind state transitions, while rapid enough to fool us, are certainly not instantaneous. They are hybrid states with qualities of both sleeping and waking that operate simultaneously. When I use the vernacular term "half awake," you know what I mean. But which part of the brain-mind is awake? Which part is lagging behind still in sleep? And how long does it really take for the lagging half to catch up?

Although they concern the most commonplace events in our daily lives, these fascinating and difficult questions are of momentous practical importance. Consider a doctor on night call in the emergency room of a busy hospital, or an air traffic controller in a large hub airport, or a radar operator on a nuclear submarine. How much disorientation can any of these people afford when many other people's lives depend upon their being at their very best?

The second part of this book examines the major faculties of the brain-mind that we depend on for life: orientation, memory, perception, emotion, attention, and energy. Each of them depends on the state the brain-mind is in. My main goal in this section is to use the brain-mind paradigm to explain how it is that these faculties work normally, and how a change in state is responsible for their going awry. All mental illnesses result from the failure of one or more of these faculties. For those who are ill, orientation gives way to disorientation, memory to confabulation, perception to hallucination, reasonable emotion to extremism, attention to distraction, and energy to despair. If a change in the state of the brain-mind can cause a faculty to fail, there is hope that we can counter mental illness by changing the state back to its rightful place (how to do so is the subject of Part Three).

Each of the next six chapters addresses one of the major faculties; in each, I intend to show how the concept of states, the AIM model, and the aminergic-cholinergic system can explain both the normal and abnormal functioning of that faculty. One of the ways to do that is to examine some of the experiences we "normal" people have. Many of us experience the symptoms of abnormal states; Delia's dreams, and mine for that matter, share many of the formal features in Bertal's psychosis. Analysis of these experiences offers strong clues to what causes an ill person to permanently harbor the symptoms that are only fleeting for us "normal" people. In chapter 12, I will then tie all these faculties together, and combine them with the paradigm developed in Part One, to create a new explanation of consciousness, unconsciousness, and the mind.

ORIENTATION: A NECESSARY TRICK

"Where am I?" is a question that we must be able to answer at every instant in time. When we are awake, we do this so effortlessly and so unconsciously that we fail to notice how important — and how active — this orientation function is in establishing our place in the world. The fact that we are so often lost in our dreams helps us appreciate the frailty of the orientation function and explains why deep study of the brain in REM sleep could give us sure clues as to how our sense of place is achieved. Other experiments of nature that result in severe disorientation, such as Alzheimer's disease, are also instructive, however cruel. How do we orient? And what state changes cause us and others to become temporarily or permanently disoriented? Let us grit our teeth and answer these questions.

Locating ourselves in space is only part of the orientation function. We also have to know who we are and what time it is.

Knowing "who we are" is not always simple. Our sense of self is a combination of internal and external monitoring, both of which are subject to failure as our brain-mind changes state over the course of each day and over a lifetime.

In many dreams neither the dreamer nor other dream characters are exactly as they should be. I often identify dream characters as persons I know only to notice that their physical features in the dream don't match up with reality. For older people, accurate identification of third persons starts to fail as memory begins to falter. This tells us that our ability to orient deteriorates with each new day, if for no other reason than that our brain cells die at an approximate rate of 50,000 per day. We need no other illness but life itself to account for a loss in orientation. Our relationships also help define who we are, and we all know how relationships can change. This is not a frivolous thought; an aging man begins to lose sight of who he is as he fails to recognize his own family members. A woman who marries happily can lose her entire sense of self when her once-trusted husband starts to beat her.

Knowing the time is not easy. A great part of the problem stems from the fact that our social world is regulated by schedules and that infernal invention, the clock. Our minds and bodies are regulated by an entirely different timer. To orient properly, we need to make a sharp distinction between external, societal time and internal, brain time. Societal time is entirely arbitrary. Our internal time is innate; when we "take our time," we proceed at a pace set by a clock inside our heads. That same clock times our moods, our drive, and our fertility.

The representations of place, time, and action in our brain-minds depend absolutely on the state our brain-minds are in. Maintaining the dramatic unities is thus much more than a theatrical nicety. In providing us with orientation, the brain-mind gives every aspect of our consciousness and our behavior their most crucial contextual dimensions. We cannot begin to evaluate anything without first correctly identifying it and locating it in place and time.

ORIENTATION AND
THE ORIENTING RESPONSE

There are two parts to our orientation faculty: an orienting response, which is our immediate reaction to an unexpected signal, and a sense of orientation, which is our ongoing assessment of place, person, and time. A quick look at what happened to me when I awoke to tinkling glasses illustrates how these two parts differ, yet work together.

When we are aroused from REM sleep and regain the orientational parameters of waking, the brain-mind must move a long distance in the three-dimensional state space that I sketched as the AIM cube. The little dot doesn't just leap instantaneously from the lower, front, right-hand corner of dreaming to the upper, back, right-hand corner of being awake. It moves there gradually, although quickly. Since the activation level (A) is already high and stays that way, any drag (or inertia) that the system must overcome during the act of waking (when we *drag* ourselves out of bed) must be due to either the information source (I) or the modulator (M). Note that during my awakening in Columbus my senses were instantly keen; my capacity to perceive the tinkling glasses was, if anything, enhanced. Thus my information-processing channels were wide open.

The most likely culprit of the inertia we must overcome during waking, then, is the modulator, the aminergic-cholinergic system. During waking, the aminergic neurons in my brain stem are resurging to take back control from the cholinergic neurons. Why should this rise be plagued by inertia? Because we need not only to get the electrical signaling of these cells up to speed (and that does happen *very* fast), but also we need to raise the concentration of their chemical products (norepinephrine and serotonin) throughout the brain. It is this wet hormonal aspect of the modulatory system that lags. Like filling a tank with fluid, it takes some time to regain full brain modulation.

My Columbus awakening story demonstrates that the orienting response happens astonishingly quickly and accurately, even though the sense of orientation takes longer to rectify. Even in my half-sleep, I could accurately localize the questionable stimulus to my right, about fifteen degrees southwest and about twenty feet away. The orienting response is a rapid reflex with little or no cognitive component. It readies our muscles for the dreaded choice: fight or flight. If the stimulus that excites such alarm later proves to be innocuous, we can simply relax; better to suppose an unknown person is a foe and later realize my mistake than ignore this possible danger and be done in.

Orientation, on the other hand, is an enduring condition and is almost wholly cognitive. Once we orient, then we begin to evaluate. This process can be complicated by emotion; because I could not quickly settle the question "who," anxiety sounded an alarm and set my fanciful thoughts in motion.

The orienting response is a reflex that has evolved to favor the fastest possible collection of the most critical external information. It is mediated by the same acetylcholine neurons of the brain stem that trigger REM sleep. The quickest way to activate "eyes right" is to buzz the nerve cells on the right side of your pons. You can't do it voluntarily as rapidly as you would if I were to clap my hands behind the right side of your head when you were not expecting a loud noise.

The orienting response is completely automatic, involuntary, and precognitive. As far as we know, it is all done unconsciously. Orientation occurs more slowly, has at least some voluntary aspects, and is cognitive. But it too is highly automatic and, at some level, I dare say, is also a quantitative computation. The computation is performed in the upper brain in response to cues perceived by the brain stem and yields answers that ground our narrative and can be retrieved in our verbal reports. But notice how closely these two processes are related: they are sequential and serial, but also simultaneous and parallel. Since both orienting and orientation depend on the brain stem and since the brain stem is chemically reorganized as we make the transition from dreaming to waking, or from any one state to another, they will both change as a function of brain-mind state, with many dramatic consequences in addition to those we have already explored.

THE MAP ROOM OF THE BRAIN

How the brain actually computes our location in space is still unknown. Evidence is accumulating to suggest that the signals derived from the orienting response may be integrated with maps that are stored in memory by a specialized brain region called the hippocampus. This map room is a specialized part of our memory bank whose contents are stored in intimate proximity to emotion central, located beside the hippocampus. The net result is that our sense of place is tied to our recollections of early experience and our sense of comfort or unease in the world.

Notice that the combination of spatial orientation, memory, and emotion that was evident in my Columbus awakening has a corresponding conjunction at the neurological level. The tying together of orienting response data (a tinkling sound to my right) with space maps stored in memory (the layout of my Boston bedroom and bathroom) and in the presence of an internal distress signal (anxiety) requires a localized brain region that is specialized to perform this three-way comparison.

If you make a fist with your right hand and tuck the end of your thumb under the forefinger, the resulting image of your hand resembles the appearance of your brain seen from above and to the left. The back of your hand and forefinger represent the cortex at the top of your brain, and your thumb represents the temporal lobe at your left ear. (The brain stem would extend directly down below the base of the palm of your hand.) The hippocampus lies approximately at your thumbnail. Alongside it in your thumb is the almond-shaped emotion factory which Latin-loving anatomists called the amygdala.

The hippocampus as map room idea has gained greater credibility through the recent work of neurophysiologists Frank Keefe and Lynn Nadel, who have found that a specific cell of the hippocampus signals most strongly as a rat moves from one specific spatial location to another. These "place-cells" must be the same ones that get turned on in our brains during REM sleep as we wander aimlessly around the landscape of our dreams.

The adjacency of our spatial memory bank (the hippocampus) and our emotion register (the amygdala) is important for both survival and procreation. Evidence is readily seen in the animal world, where knowing who else is in one's territory (friend? foe? mate?) and knowing what behavior is appropriate (fight or flight? approach or avoid?) really matters.

The question, then, is whether our own altered brain-mind states, and especially our dreams, aren't reminding us of just how important all of this place, person, and time knowledge really is. Why else would the brain-mind expend so much of its cognitive effort at trying, in vain, to settle on a reliable dream locale, to establish a consistent cast of dream characters, and to situate the action in a particular time period. In this sense, Freud was right: dreams are trying to tell us something important about our instincts (sex, aggression), our feelings (fear, anger, affection), and our lives (places, persons, and times). From studying waking, sleeping, and dreaming, we can, therefore, derive a theory of how these crucial life data are programmed, integrated, and maintained using one of our most fundamental faculties — orientation. A closer look at some of the orientational factors of Delia's dreams will show how they coincide with instinct and emotion.

CREATING THE BIZARRENESS OF DREAMS

Through an extensive set of observations of many reports, my sleep lab group has established the surprising and previously unrecognized fact that most of what we consider to be the strangeness of dreams derives from their orientational instability. As we have seen, dreams — with all their wonderfully cathartic dramas — not only flagrantly violate Aristotle's canonical unities of time, place and action but also often confound the identities of the actors.

To illustrate orientational instability let's look again at Delia's first dream, the one in which she was flying in the balloon with her father and sisters, then landed in Paris-by-the-sea, saw the boy pissing in the water, and ended up planning her visit to the Al-Aqsa Mosque. The way that we score the dream is to underline the phrases in Delia's dream report that portray instances of "bizarreness." Bizarreness is defined as improbable details of either the dream plot or the dreamer's thoughts and feelings. For each bizarre item that is identified in a report, we next try to situate the item — was it in the plot itself or in the dreamer's thoughts or feelings? Finally, we determine whether the bizarreness quality of the item stemmed from discontinuity, incongruity, or uncertainty.

What results is a table listing the relative frequency of each bizarreness category. Delia's balloon dream was typical in that the three leading bizarrenesses identified were plot incongruity, plot discontinuity, and cognitive uncertainty. You too could return to my hotel dream or my summary of Delia's balloon dream report and score it for yourself to get the hang of it; you may even want to record some dreams of your own and score them using the technique. What you will end up with is a list that is structured like this:

Bizarre item	Situated	Quality
It seemed to become a live aerial view	Plot	Discontinuity
Down to the seashore (Paris was on the North Sea)	Plot	Incongruity
I saw a young boy peeing in the water	Plot	Incongruity

Plot Incongruity

Far and away the most common peculiarity of Delia's dream, and all dreams, is that the characters, settings, and actions have mismatched or otherwise inappropriate features. Sometimes these represent physical impossibilities like the map that suddenly becomes an aerial view, but usually they are more subtle, such as when she said that she walked down to the seashore or saw the Al-Aqsa Mosque. This class of items seems to reflect a kind of overinclusiveness, as if the reference files for a given item — such as "Delia's tourism" — were more wide open than is permitted in waking. The associative rules are so loosened that almost anything fits into a dream scenario.

Plot Discontinuity

Less common, but no less distinctive, is a sudden change in the identity or characteristics of a person, a place, or an action. The Paris city map that metamorphoses into a live aerial view is a striking case in point. More dramatic discontinuities can segment the plot into entirely separate scenes by changing all facets of orientation at once. This class of item would seem to reflect the activation of cognitive schemata and their neuronal network infrastructure. The new schematic networks might or might not be associated with the ones they have replaced. While it is generally assumed that the successive scenes of a dream deal with a single, unifying theme, we will later consider persuasive evidence that even thematic unity is sometimes flagrantly violated.

Cognitive Uncertainty

The second most common item to be scored as bizarre by waking standards is explicit vagueness regarding orientational details; such vagueness may be expressed whether or not the items themselves are bizarre. Delia's balloon dream does not illustrate this feature dramatically, but her use of the phrase "seemed to" in describing the transmogrification of the Paris city map into the live aerial view comes close to it. Whether this class of item is convincingly bizarre is debatable. I include it because it is so prevalent in many dream reports and because I find it odd that in my own dreams I can't either coherently imagine well-known characters or be sure of the identity of some characters that are clearly imagined. Both the perceptual assemblies (the images) and their nominal attributes (their names) tend to be unaccountably peculiar. If I had these two difficulties in my waking life, my orientational capability would be grossly defective.

MICRO BIZARRENESS, MACRO STABILITY

All the items described in the bizarreness inventory are relatively detailed. At a higher level of dream organization, the spatial locations are stable for each of the four scenes. Indeed, it is this stability that defines what we mean by a "scene." Furthermore, the dream loci are stable in ways that we must consider to be significant with respect to the dreamer's goals and life history.

Scene 1 takes place in the balloon, an exotic setting reflecting Delia's lifelong desire to transcend mundane reality. But her father and sisters are also in this perilous craft with her. Something (fear?) is pulling them down, but this in turn obviates the need to end the trip.

Here we see the way in which Delia's orientational instability interacts with her deep motivational drives. Into the holes and spaces of her defective dream cognition flow the hopes, wishes, and fears that are tied to the key drives in her life. The sense and the nonsense of her dream are two sides of the same coin. It is this reciprocal aspect that has led me to call dreaming a physiological Rorschach test. Like the meaningless ink blots that Hermann Rorschach asked his patients to identify, the REM-sleep brain sends itself senseless electrical messages and says, "Tell me what you see!" The resulting dream reflects our innate tendency to project meaning onto stimuli. What we see, feel, and do in our dreams reveals our specific and personal predilections. I should point out, however, that by using this analogy, I do not scientifically endorse the practice or the interpretive accuracy of either the Rorschach test or any particular sort of dream analysis. Interpretation is always a risky, speculative enterprise.

Delia doesn't have to go home, after all. She can stay in Paris and continue her quest for exotic adventures on firm ground. So the beat goes on, at least for Delia, and in Scene 2 she explores the city and finds the seashore to visit, where she goes wading. We assume her father and sisters are still there but they are not mentioned again. But again she is blocked. Delia is like the nursery rhyme girl who asks her mother if she can go out to swim and is told, "Yes, my darling daughter. Hang your clothes on a hickory limb but don't go near the water!" A boy is urinating and so polluting her bathing place.

In Scenes 3 and 4 she is still questing, but now her goal is the Al-Aqsa Mosque. This is exotic enough, surely, but notice that her plan to visit this holy place of Islam is now sanctified by prayer, by worship. Her quest for adventure has now been tamed, neutralized, and socialized. She is a good girl after all. Only in seeking directions to the mosque from the lady behind the hotel desk does she once again "take off," but this time it is entirely via the visualization of the aerial view of Paris, which serves her need to find the mosque entrance so she can say her morning prayers.

Looking at the dream in this way emphasizes the clarity and coherence of its structure. Overriding the microscopic bizarreness, which I am inclined to discount as meaningless brain-mind noise, is the manifestly coherent narrative that displays, with limpid clarity, many of Delia's psychological concerns. By discounting dream bizarreness as noise, we are freed from any interpretive obligation to it and can instead focus our attention on the directly relevant nature of this dream's content.

This way of sorting dream wheat from chaff runs counter to classical psychoanalytic practice. Because Freud thought that dreams were most meaningful when they appeared most crazy, he was inspired to posit a censor that disguised the dream data so that it could not possibly be understood without interpretation via free association. Our new theory allows us to dispense with Freud's distinction between the manifest content (which he demeaned and we consider valuable) and the latent content (which he extolled and we consider noise).

The related dream characters, settings, and emotions are read out as Delia's hippocampus and amygdala are stimulated by her brain stem. On top of these stable plots is a jumble of cognitive oddities, which implies that the brain-mind cannot achieve full coherence of dream plot detail because there are too many unpredictable and irrelevant stimuli emanating from Delia's brain stem. The failure to achieve tight coherence of dream plot may also be due to chemical demodulation of Delia's cortex, which contains the information needed to round out the dream scenario in an internally consistent way.

Put another way, Delia's brain-mind calls upon its own records of significant places, people, relationships, and feelings to achieve such order as is possible under the curiously altered conditions of the dream state. While this could be taken to mean that dreams reveal unconscious mental structures not otherwise available to the subject, that is not necessarily so. As we have just seen in the last few paragraphs, the same information is readily available from Delia during her waking state. There was no need for a Freudian exploration into her unconscious; all the information was easily accessible when simply talking to Delia.

What is most dreamy about dreams? What is most strange? Discontinuity, incongruity, and uncertainty. These are all disruptions in orientation. They are all problems of place, person, and time. Of all the impressive features of Delia's dreams, and mine and yours and everyone's, orientational instability is the most fundamental. The reason for this is that the dream state is different from the waking state. Dreaming is an organic psychosis, and the other instances when we see orientation as a problem are the other organic psychoses — when the brain cells of an Alzheimer's patient are dying, or the brain cells of an alcoholic are pickled. During dreaming there is no death of cells, no drug, but there is a physical cause for the disorientation; the amines — the norepinephrine or serotonin — are nowhere to be found. Acetylcholine has swept them out. And so we see how the brain-mind paradigm explains orientation during waking, and disorientation during dreaming, that healthy psychosis.

But what of Bertal? If the brain-mind paradigm holds true, then a similar explanation should hold for Bertal's episodes of hallucination. And indeed it does.

As it is for Delia's dreams, disorientation is a fundamental trait of Bertal's psychotic episodes. Clearly, he was disoriented when he envisioned dive-bombers coming at him at The Psycho. His mind could not even begin to justify dive-bombers as real unless he was severely disoriented, because he was *inside a building* at the time of the "raid." Disorientation also led to his attack on me in my office. He thought he was in a "house of peace and rest" because he saw white walls, heard a solemn quiet, felt hard floors beneath his feet; that's why he knelt at my office door and genuflected. Then he saw me standing there, in a white doctor's coat, which by this point, to his mind, could be readily mistaken for a holy robe, and he therefore mistook me for Jesus or God. His mind was doing the exact same thing that Delia's was: receiving images and imposing a scenario that "made sense" out of them, in order to try to orient him — to tell him where he was and who the people were around him. The difference, since he was awake, was that his motor impulses were not inhibited and he was indeed able to kneel and lunge at me. Why he lunged is another question, but why he thought I was a holy man in the first place was the result of disorientation.

DISORIENTATION
IN DIFFERENT STATES

We can better understand the faculty of orientation by looking at the orienting response and its counterpart, habituation. Like the boy who cried wolf too often, handclaps — even thunderclaps — lose their power to make us jump if they occur frequently enough.

Since the orienting reaction, with its rapid redirection of our eyes and our heads, is a reflex, the capacity to diminish the orienting response is also automatic. But how can an automatic system "know" how to recognize a stimulus as familiar? When a surprising signal, like the sharp report of a firecracker, enters the brain stem, it catches the neurons napping. As a motor response is being prepared, the "Where is it?" orienting signals are sent into the upper brain to prepare those networks for the analytic task of determining the significance of the stimulus.

Under conditions of sustained threat, the orientation system considers every sound as dangerous. During the bombing of London in World War II, British citizens hiding in underground shelters considered every enginelike sound to be that of a German airplane. When Khrushchev was found to have installed missiles in Cuba — and Kennedy learned that more were on the way — we Americans were faced with the realistic threat of being bombarded for the first time since World War II. I vividly remember the mass startle response of thirty scientists in 1962 when a loud explosion suddenly interrupted our night course in calculus at the National Institutes of Health near Washington. We were all under our desks before our orientation system recognized that the source of the sound was a car backfiring, and not one of Castro's missiles blowing up the Pentagon!

The brain-stem signals that prepare the upper-brain networks for their analytic task of asking "What is it?" include messages from the acetylcholine neurons. These brain-stem signals are so strong they can actually be recorded as prominent waves in the EEG, called "evoked potentials," of an animal that is startled during waking. This internal communication system utilizes acetylcholine, and although it is not yet exactly clear why, the current thinking is that acetylcholine may act as a chemical exclamation point. It reinforces the significance of other signals coming into the visual brain by saying, "Hey, you'd better sit up and take notice of this image!"

The first wave of any series of extreme stimuli causes the release of a large amount of acetylcholine. It also excites the serotonin neurons, which, as we already know, put a damper on the cholinergic system. But the serotonin effect is delayed and prolonged. It does not diminish the first response, but it does suppress the response to subsequent stimuli, each of which keeps the damper on as long as they are repeated frequently enough to guarantee their familiarity. If I enter the room when my partner is working intently, he will jump and admit severe fright despite his prompt recognition that it is only me. But once startled, his vulnerability to a repeat performance is markedly diminished. I couldn't scare him if I tried. He becomes habituated.

It would thus seem that our state-control system is also an elemental learning machine, since it knows how to change its responses based on its experience. But now we need to ask, "Suppose it changes state. What happens to its knowledge then?"

Because the motor aspects of the startle reflex are suppressed in REM, our brain-mind needs some other outlet for reactions to stimuli. During our dreams we constantly invent imaginary interlopers in response to the acetylcholine and electrical stimuli entering our cortex. Bertal does the same.

It is in this sense that we are repeatedly surprised by unexpected events, by strange people, by feelings of alarm, and by the full bag of orientational tricks that our brain-mind employs when it lacks external space-time cues. Our capacity to get used to being lost is itself lost. So everything seems novel, seizes our interest, absorbs us totally, and makes us feel wholly engaged in the fool's errand of finding out where we are, who else is there, and what is going on. In dreamland, it is a blind-man's bluff, it is hide-and-seek from start to finish. And, as in these children's games, we are always "it."

MY LOST MOTHER

In our dreams, we experience the brain-mind state of so many of our fellow humans who suffer from mental illness, those unfortunates who are always "it," always looking for something that is not there and often unaware that they are caught in a vicious game of hide-and-seek. Put more harshly, when we dream we are being treated to a preview of coming distractions, those that age and degeneration of our own brain-minds may bring. Now that we know the chemistry of how the brain-mind becomes disoriented, however, we may be able to apply it to mental illness.

When my mother became lost during a game of bridge, I should have caught on. She had always been such a good bridge player that I failed to understand her strange behavior one night when I first noticed her spatial disorientation. It was in July 1977, and we had taken a small house in an abandoned Italian village near Pisa in Tuscany. Every Monday I drove a perilous mule trail down to Bagni di Lucca and then on to Pisa to collect a trunkful of books for my research on *The Dreaming Brain*. The rest of the week I worked in the morning, enjoyed exploratory trips with my family in the afternoon, and in the evening, after dinner, sat with them all in the kitchen to play bridge.

My mother, who was then seventy-three, and I were on one team, and my wife and son were on the other. I had first bid spades, and my mother and I took the contract at four. As is usual, I invited my mother to display her trump cards, the spades, before my son led the first card of the hand. She laid down a very nice set of spades, but to my astonishment she placed them in a column to her left and not to her right, as convention dictates.

When I thoughtlessly blurted out my objection she was quite insistent. With her characteristic deference and sweetness she said, "I always put them down on this side." I still didn't get it. As a result of my increasing obstinacy, she finally gave in, saying, "Oh, have it your way," and changed the trump file from her left to her right. We went on to win the rubber as she played her subsequent hand with her usual skill.

But then, when we were on an outing in Florence, my mother

had trouble remembering where she had parked the car. This was easy enough to dismiss on a hot summer day in a foreign city full of short-tempered tourists like ourselves. And dismiss it we did. It was not until the next fall when a policeman found her confused and utterly lost on a back road near her own house in New Hampshire that the lights finally went on in our heads and we realized there was something sadly amiss in the map room of her mind.

In retrospect, I'm glad it took us so long to realize that she had begun to undergo that inexorable degeneration of brain cells named after the Munich psychiatrist Alois Alzheimer. As a result, she had half a year of freedom and we had six more months of enjoyment of her company without any contemplation of the pain that lay ahead.

The most confounding feature of Alzheimer's is disorientation. And although brain scientists don't yet know how to fit all the pieces together, it is becoming clear that Alzheimer's is almost entirely the result of a problem in brain chemistry. The brain-mind paradigm offers us some hope.

It seems quite likely that in Alzheimer's disease *both* the acetylcholine and serotonin systems suffer from the widespread loss of cells. The sleep architecture of Alzheimer's patients is as topsyturvy as their memory when they are awake. Alzheimer's is a disease of structure that affects all the states of the brain-mind.

Those of us with a healthy complement of brain cells are more likely to become disoriented around the edges of sleep. One way to gain insight into Alzheimer's, then, is to further study what happens to us as we make the transition from waking to sleeping and back again. The capacity of our brain-mind to attend, to remember, and to control emotion is decidedly diminished at the edges of sleep. I daresay these important functions slide imperceptibly but significantly all day long. Why else do most of us work most effectively in the morning? The most logical answer is because we've just slept and these functions have had a chance to restore themselves.

The current theory is that our faculties function best in the morning because the ratio of aminergic to cholinergic neurotransmission is maximal at that time. Put another way, we are at the top of the modulatory (M) axis in the AIM model. We are sharp, interested, attentive, and effective at our data-processing tasks. As the day moves on, the aminergic system loses its edge and the cholinergic system escapes tight control. Our mental lapses first increase in frequency and finally become continuous when it is time for lights-out.

In sleep, what had been a slow decline becomes a slippery slope. As aminergic activity plummets, cholinergic activity surges. Now, in our dreams, we can see things that aren't there, believe things that aren't true, become completely disoriented, explain away our demented state by concocting wild stories, and then — conveniently perhaps — forget our nocturnal madness.

As for the purpose of this flimflam, we imagine that our aminergic brain cells might benefit from their time off. Perhaps they are able to restore their chemical power by building new molecules and not having to use them. At the same time, our cholinergic neurons are having a field day, so they become tamed and more easily managed by the time we wake up in the morning. What's more, their rambunctious activity overnight could have tuned our brain circuits by running them in the dark, in essence using our dreams as test programs. To take but one example — that of orientation — it seems possible that we get lost in dreams in order to stay found in waking.

The changes in our faculties that so closely parallel changes in our brain state should convince us all of the virtues of the brain-mind paradigm. Whether it be over the course of a day or over the course of a lifetime, it is in the structure and function of our neurons that we find the most fundamental ways of understanding our extraordinary talent for orientation (and as we will see in subsequent chapters, for memory, and attention, and other faculties as well).

In fact, we can now see why we called the brightest students in our high school and college classes "brains." Their prodigious feats of memorization, their speed in perceiving the logic of a geometry theorem or the allegorical significance of a short story, their uncanny ability to concentrate on their homework — all these mental skills were manifestations of optimal brain-mind state control.

These brainy kids were the paragons of the brain-mind paradigm. Their superb cerebral hardware was a fortuitous genetic accident. Their versatile mental software was a great programming job done in the childhood and teenage environments of their lives, which loaded and fine-tuned their cerebral circuits for efficient and accurate processing both on-line and off.

CHAPTER 7

The Story of Our Lives:
Memory and Confabulation

N THE 1960s, many people in the psychoanalytic community believed that our lives were the enactment of scripts prewritten into our minds. Now most psychoanalysts contend that we write our own scripts as we go along, pulling up old scenes to help us navigate through new ones. Those old scenes are our memories. And as Freud himself insisted, it's not what really has happened to us that matters — it's our recollection of what has happened that matters.

Any parent knows what this means. As parents try to advance a relationship with their child, they look back to how their own parents interacted with them. What they are calling up, however, is not what actually happened, but their *recollection* of what happened.

We all do this. There is no alternative. During Christmas I am always reminded of how, when I was a small boy, I looked up the chimney to see if Santa Claus was real. Whether I actually remember doing that, at such a young age, or am remembering the story my parents always told me of my doing it, I can't say. It's our reconstruction of early events, our *fantasy* about them, that operates in our minds today.

My Santa Claus myth connotes precocious scientific skepticism. We all manage our daily lives, our important relationships, and our emotional upheavals by means of stories that we tell ourselves about ourselves. We are all our own PR agents. At the highest level of our consciousness, there is a set of precepts, explanations, and rules without which we would be unable to cope with life. We constantly try to clarify and articulate what these important representations actually are, and then we make a deliberate effort to create alternative descriptions of ourselves so that we can live our lives more happily. We all constantly elaborate narrative structures to explain and guide our behavior. Some of the material is historical truth, and some of it is pure fiction. And some of it may just be made up on the spot to suit the need of our current script.

What are memories? There are no words, no sentences, no pictures, no stories in our heads, any more than there are sentences in the word processor that records this manuscript, flashes it up on a screen, and then prints it out on paper. There are only bits of data. Our memories exist as groupings of data in the activated neuronal networks of our brain-mind. Visual images, maps of space, and motor programs are all produced when we activate the appropriate network.

Memory itself is not a thing. It is a process of neuronal network activation. Sometimes we are immediately able to activate the network, say, to recall the name of a person we know we should know, and sometimes we can't. Some memory networks self-activate in perpetuity, no matter how useless the information. The telephone number of my childhood home, which I left over forty years ago, is 232–0043; on the last day of the baseball season in 1944, Snuffy Stirnweiss of the New York Yankees lost the American League batting championship to Luke Appling of the Chicago White Sox by a few thousandths of a percentage point. I still remember crying as I did the long division to figure out the result (I was a Yankee fan). Other networks last only a few days and are gone: what did you eat for dinner last Monday?

Memories are strongly dependent on the state of the brain-mind. When I enter REM sleep each night and the modulatory chemistry of my brain changes its state, I am liable to recall ex-

traordinarily remote memories. Recently my sixth-grade classmate
Dick Tinguely suddenly popped into one of my dreams after a fifty-
two-year absence from any other aspect of my conscious experience. Funny to think of Dick lying quietly in a furrow of my brain
for all those years. Just as Dick Tinguely pops up during my dream,
acquaintances long forgotten pop up during yours. Yet, as we have
already seen, we rarely remember a dream we had just a few hours,
or even minutes, earlier. People who can put themselves in a trance
can suddenly hear the voice of their mother or father, deceased
for years. The morning after a night of drunkenness, they can't
remember what they did.

All these odd traits of memory are only beginning to be understood. How does memory work? Why does it change with state?
How can it leave us, and those with mental illnesses, temporarily or
permanently? Let us use the brain-mind model to work out some
preliminary answers.

THAT CAR LOOKS LIKE
IT'S BEEN IN AN ACCIDENT

I was standing on the sidewalk in front of a nineteenth-century
apartment house on the Quai Aristide Briand in Lyon, France,
when the narrative networks of my brain emitted an ominous an-
nouncement: That car looks like it's been in an accident. And indeed, the rear end of the English Riley 1.5 parked next to the curb
was a mess — as if some other car had driven into it at considerable speed. The crowd of passersby that had gathered to survey
the wreck, and discuss its possible cause in heated Gallic debate,
indicated that the accident must have been recent. It was hard for
me to tell, exactly, because I had trouble understanding their
French. Then I had a very alarming thought.

However damaged, that looks like my car. But it couldn't be, I
told myself. There is nothing wrong with my car. Then I noticed
that down the road about a hundred yards was a small blue French
Renault with a bridge abutment sticking up through its hood like
the Eiffel Tower. Another crowd of garrulous and gesticulating

Frenchmen was trying to extricate the driver from the crumpled front seat of that vehicle.

I wonder how the driver of this car [referring to the one that looked like mine] is doing? I asked myself. He must be okay, because there is no one in the car and there is no one lying on the sidewalk.

A member of the argumentative crowd that had gathered around the car before me then asked me some questions that I couldn't understand well enough to respond. I just smiled helplessly as I usually do when at a loss in a foreign country — or a strange situation — and that seemed to satisfy the group. They went back to gesticulating and, as I gathered from their gestures, to arguing about what had happened and who might have been at fault. By this time a policeman had arrived, as well as an ambulance that emitted a terrifying honk instead of a siren.

I looked at the car again.

Practically totaled, I concluded. I'm glad it just looks like mine. Amazing coincidence. Black (just like mine), cute little English four-seater (just like mine), red leather bucket seats (just like mine), walnut dashboard (just like mine). Riley 1.5, rare make (just like mine). Extremely difficult to repair, said my narrative network.

All the features of the wreck matched those of my own car. Even the license plate, Rhode Island, MD 353, which could be seen in the crumpled folds of the bashed trunk, matched those of my vehicle. I was surprised by all these details but was at something of a loss to understand how such coincidences could be explained.

Yet I wasn't disoriented. I knew who I was. I knew it was Saturday, October 9, 1963. And I even knew that I was standing on the sidewalk of the Quai Aristide Briand, which runs alongside the Rhône River. I promptly recognized my wife, Joan, when she shouldered her way through the crowd and asked me, "Are you okay?"

"Okay? Of course I'm okay. But look at that car. What a mess! Glad it's not ours. It just looks like ours," I reassured her.

"But it *is* our car," she asserted, "and when I went into the house to pick up the baby-sitter, you were sitting in the driver's seat."

"Oh yes," I said, without any real conviction and promptly forgot what I had just been told.

"From the baby-sitter's apartment above I heard the crash," she continued. "Some drunk ran into you from behind. Both his legs are broken!"

"How dreadful" was the best I could do for him. I could see that he had been extricated from his car and was about to be whisked off to the hospital by the mournfully honking ambulance.

Since my wife had identified me as the driver of the stove-in Riley, the policeman was now asking me a lot of questions. But I was not giving him what he wanted. "Too bad he doesn't speak French as well as you, madame," he said to my wife (in French, of course).

"But his French is usually fluent," Joan told him. "There must be something wrong with his head. He can't seem to remember anything."

Joan's diagnosis didn't slow the gendarme down any. He and the sidewalk jury all agreed with me that I was fine. "*N'inquietez vous*," he said, meaning, "Not to worry."

But I did have some concern about our one-year-old son. "How is Ian?" I asked.

"Fine," Joan said. "He is at home."

I still had enough self-reflective awareness to realize I could not form a record of my frightening experience. I did not have enough memory to make a lasting, useful set of representations of my extremely perilous state or even to create a story explaining what had caused me to be so dim. And in my insistence that I was fine, I really thought I was fine. I wasn't deliberately confabulating either.

Meanwhile, the gendarme was behaving with a bureaucratic thoroughness that matched his medical incompetence. We would be well advised to call a *huissier,* the gendarme kept saying. Neither Joan nor I, at our best, knew that *huissier* was the French equivalent of "justice of the peace," a public official whose documentation of a serious accident is required by insurance companies, especially when there has been severe bodily injury. The baby-sitter's mother not only translated this rare French word but called up a live one on the telephone.

Before this worthy's arrival — and no more than ten minutes after my memory had been blasted out of that bucket seat — I began to feel distinctly woozy. I don't recall whether the lights went all the way out, but I was suddenly on my back on the sidewalk.

Before long, I too was laid out in an ambulance. With Joan riding shotgun, the ambulance honked and careened along the quai toward the emergency room of the Grange Blanche Hospital. The hospital actually sits right across the Boulevard Rockefeller from the medical school in Lyon where I had been studying the control of conscious states by the brain stem. I was scared. I knew I had amnesia and I knew I was in shock. The "onk-onk" of the ambulance seemed to go straight to the anxiety center in my brain, which responded by sending back rhythmic waves of panic.

Yet I was *not* disoriented. I could more or less visualize the whole ambulance trip on the map of Lyon in my mind. And in the emergency ward, when I found that I could sit if not stand, I was even able to help Joan and the intern get through the mental status exam! But I still couldn't give them a history of the accident. I had no recent memory. I could formulate no propositions about the recent past. And even though I was a doctor and a brain specialist, I could offer no explanation about why I was amnesic. Although the honking had stopped, I still felt scared.

Despite my objections, the doctors decided to admit me for observation. I hate hospitals, at least when I'm the patient. And I felt pretty sure that I was already getting better. My French was coming back. I even remembered going out to dinner the night before and that we were headed for a rugby game when I got clobbered outside the baby-sitter's house. And — last of all — I remembered that my cousin George was coming the next evening with a promise to take us to dinner at Fernand Point's La Pyramide Restaurant in nearby Vienne. I wasn't going to miss that one even if I was delirious.

But I had to admit that I still couldn't remember the accident at all. Joan had to keep telling me about it and reassuring me about Ian. So before she left to go home to take care of him, she wrote me a narrative script that could serve as a stand-in for my lost memory.

The observation ward in which I lay was not comforting. The man in the bed next to mine was comatose and gurgling. To rule out the supposition that I too might be dying, I read my script, which said: "You've been in an accident."

"The car is badly damaged."

"Ian is fine."

"I am fine [meaning Joan]."

"The guy in the next bed is in much worse shape than you are!"

It worked for long enough to let me doze. Then I was awakened by the gurgling from the next bed. And again I read the script. And again I slept.

This cycle repeated itself throughout the evening until I finally fell into a long and deep sleep. By morning, when the neurologists made their rounds, I really *was* fine. My mental status exam was normal: I was oriented to time, place, and person; my recent memory was intact; and my emotions were stable. My blood pressure was normal. The formulation of the events of the accident, and its effect on my brain-mind, which the French doctors and I made together — in French — was crystal clear. Here is the formulation we elaborated:

I was sitting in the driver's seat of my Riley 1.5 waiting for my wife to come downstairs with the baby-sitter we were picking up to take care of Ian, so we could go to a rugby game.

I was double-parked on a road on which people often speed, and I could remember nervously eyeing the rearview mirror. Although there were two other free lanes between me and the Rhône River, I was astonished to see the ever-enlarging image of a Renault weaving its way toward me. Paralyzed with fear, and having inadequate time to move my car or jump out of it, I was struck from behind and my car was violently accelerated forward. But since inertia held most of me still, my head snapped backward as the bucket seat shot forward against my back. It was whiplash at its worst.

The mental image of a snapping whip helped the doctors and me visualize the sudden S-shaped deformation my brain stem underwent when my head first snapped back away from my body when the car was hit, then rebounded forward again as the car rapidly decelerated and stopped. My head probably didn't move farther than a foot and a half off its usual vertical alignment with my body, and since there was no evidence of any impact to my head on either its backward or forward flight, we assumed, simply, that my brain stem, the soft spongy bit of tissue that makes me breathe and dream, was just twisted and tugged a whole lot more than it likes to be.

If I had hit my head on the steering wheel, the amnesia that I suffered would have been easy to explain. In such a case the temporal lobes are jostled by an effect called contre-coup (meaning "against the blow"). This is what happens to a boxer whose head is rocked back so fast by a knockout punch that it leaves his brain behind; his brain crashes into the front wall of his skull. After too many such bouts a boxer's memory may leave him for good.

Even though my head hit nothing, my brain may have crashed against the front wall of my skull as the car rapidly decelerated. That entirely internal impact may have added the insult of temporal lobe concussion to the injury of brain-stem whiplash.

Considering that I was able to recover so quickly, my brain was probably not even bruised. What really happened to my brain that day I will never know, which is too bad because it could tell me a lot. In addition to the sudden and dramatic amnesia about the accident, I had a partial loss of many representations of the previous months. Most strikingly, my hard-earned fluency in French had temporarily disappeared.

Until my blood pressure took a dive on the sidewalk, and I with it, we assumed that whatever went wrong was mainly neuronal. I supposed that the tug caused some local changes in blood supply so that the neurons were temporarily short of oxygen or were perhaps bathed in a slight but suddenly quite different concentration of salt. I also wondered if the modulatory neurons on which I depended to hold data in working memory might have decreased their output below a critical level. To anyone who wanted to know what was going on, I was suddenly about as useful as a cabbage.

The rest of my brain was actually fine, however, so I had gotten out of the car, walked around to what used to be its rear end, and said to myself, That car looks like it's been in an accident.

The Grange Blanche neurologists agreed with my theory about my state, but they weren't about to let me leave the hospital until they had run a lot of tests. They naturally wanted to protect themselves — and me I suppose — from the oversight of some alternative explanation. But I still wanted out. So I said that since my lab colleagues at the medical school were all neurologists, I would be under constant surveillance. And I agreed to sign a release and to get all the tests done as an outpatient.

They still didn't look happy. So I played my trump card, my cousin's dinner invitation. When they heard I was going to La Pyramide and that someone else was going to be paying the bill, they all smiled at each other with gastronomic glee and said, "*Va-t-on*," meaning, "Beat it." I shall never forget that dinner!

MEMORY, REMEMBERING, AND LEARNING

A memory itself is unobservable. It is stored as a pattern of electrical sequences in the brain. Remembering is an act — the activation of that electrical sequence. When we remember, we call up a word, a phone number, or a recipe and hold it in consciousness, or project it as a visual image on the screen that we call our mind's eye.

Memories can be implicit or explicit. Implicit memory involves only recognition; an aging woman can show through emotions that she knows someone even though she cannot recall their name. Explicit memory involves active recall. Almost all memory is completely unconscious almost all the time. Memory is unconscious even when it is revealing itself clearly in elaborate and overlearned behaviors, like playing the piano or speaking. When we perform such acts, we are not aware of accessing memory at all — how to move our fingers or our tongues. They just move. We may become conscious of the role of memory, but only after the fact. This so-called procedural memory is relatively automatic, like motor patterns.

So where are memories stored when we are not remembering them? Not in some neatly localized file. Very recent research indicates they are represented in neuronal activity patterns that are widely distributed throughout the brain; one piece of evidence to support this notion is that procedural memory in people and animals is not eliminated when damage occurs to any particular part of the brain.

When we want to retrieve a name from memory, then, the task is not a matter of finding its location. It is a matter of turning on its representation. We know this intuitively; if we try too hard to search for a lost name, we may actually impede its retrieval. We say, ironically, "If I forget about it, it will come to me." And lo and behold it does. Why not store a memory in just one place? One answer may be redundancy. Just as most of us keep copies of the computer programs on our hard drives on a floppy disk, in case an electrical misadventure causes our computer to crash, our brain does the same. You can have a small localized stroke and not lose your memory.

There is a more positive reason for storing memories in a distributed way, too. It makes us more versatile in associating data with as many contexts and skills as possible. Since it is not always obvious what contexts are likely to be relevant in the future, it is useful to associate some new piece of data with all the possible contexts of its relevance.

When I first bought my old dairy farm in Vermont, I was appalled at all the junk the previous owners had accumulated. Cursing their laziness, I tore into the unsightly scrap metal heaps that cluttered the shed and fields alike. You've probably seen those old automobile carcasses sprouting petunias, wagons disguised by weeds, ancient hay rakes enmeshed in burdock, and tangled fence rolls trailing morning glory. Such rubbish was the bane of a city-bred fixer-upper. Grunting, sweating, and self-satisfied, I threw them all out.

Then I tackled the drainage problem behind the barn. My

In REM sleep, the amines, which function as the C neurons, have retreated. But when we wake up they return. Every A-B excitation is again associated with an input from the C cells. So now the information is more likely to be retained in memory. Why do we remember any dreams at all? Because the activated neurons that represent the dream plot are only relatively demodulated (they are not gone), and because upon our waking their influence may rise rapidly enough to cement the otherwise transitory dream excitation into the form of a memory. Many neurobiologists now believe that the modulatory neurons confer some permanent structural change on the brain cells that they contact and that this change constitutes the same fundamental mechanism of learning and memory at all levels of the animal kingdom, from snails to humans.

MANAGING MEMORY

If we have to be awake to remember, what could be the memory function of dreaming? Do we dream to somehow strengthen memory? Do we dream in order to forget? We're not sure, but the one psychological quality that is maintained in every definition of dreaming over the centuries is that it is hyperassociative; the categories that we link when we dream are so broad they become over-inclusive.

All of which implies that I don't dream of axles because they symbolically represent beams, or phalluses for that matter. I dream of axles, beams, phalluses, and whatever else because they are associated in some (or several) broad categories. One function of my dream might thus be to associate my memories and so increase their versatility and redundancy. A wagon axle is also a probe, a battering ram, a crowbar, and a drill — it can poke, hit, pry, and screw. To be usable, its representation should be stored in all those categories so as to be easily accessible from all of them.

I believe, though I can't yet prove it, that the brain-mind traverses the states of non-REM and REM sleep in part to reinforce and reorganize memory. Reinforcement occurs via consolidation: an experience that we had during the day is represented as an A-B connection temporarily enhanced by a C chemical (like norepinephrine or serotonin). In sleep the brain changes the status of that sensitized connection from temporary to permanent by removing the C chemical and adding a D chemical (like acetylcholine).

Though still speculation, there is mounting evidence that one of the reasons we need sleep at all is to permanently encode our memories. We sleep, and the past day's memories are reactivated as we dream, which changes their status; it advances them from short-term memory into long-term memory, perhaps by imposition of acetylcholine, which is omnipresent during sleep.

A colleague of mine related a story about his college housemate's peculiar study habit. The housemate was an accounting major and therefore had to commit to memory large stores of numbers, formulas, and case studies each day. When it came time to study he would retreat to his sparsely furnished bedroom and recline on his bed, propping his head up with a pillow against the wall. He would open an accounting book and read intently for forty-five minutes to an hour, scribbling in the margins when necessary. He would then doze off, for no more than fifteen minutes but no less than five. He would awake, resume another hour of work, then doze off again. The pattern repeated itself three or four times each evening (unless there was a good party, of course). His nocturnal sleep schedule was no different from that of any other college student. He never expressed mental fatigue, yet was usually unaware that he was dozing off, retorting to my colleague's taunts that he had just closed his eyes for a minute.

Was the housemate's brain shutting down to sift information once the funnel was full, to store what was useful and drain off the rest, emptying the funnel for the next load? This is just conjecture, but it is possible. The housemate was a brilliant student and didn't nap under any other circumstances. Thomas Edison, whom we will meet again later in this book, glorified the "power nap" and its capacity to fuel inventiveness. By nodding off for a quick five under the stairs of his Menlo Park laboratory, Edison may have been using his REM sleep not only to store but to recombine creatively his ideational data.

The instances of letting the brain shut down in order to process information are all around us. When we have a vexing problem, our friends tell us to sleep on it, and the matter does seem simpler come morning. Writers who have written themselves into dead ends are told by their editors to put the draft in a drawer for the weekend, and a pathway out usually does present itself come Monday morning. Children, when they must memorize a list of facts for school, are often found with their eyes closed repeating the list to themselves over and over. Though it is not sleep, it has some of the same effects; they are putting themselves into a mild trance with the mnemonic mantra and relieving the brain of external stimuli so it can encode the devilish list.

In addition to consolidation, changing the status of what is remembered during sleep could have three other purposes. The representation of the memory in neuronal networks could be made more secure by its simultaneous distribution to other networks. It could be made more versatile by linking it in hyperassociative fashion to every network with which it shares formal features (such as axles with long things, hard things, strong things). It could be made more useful if it were linked to procedures that it served (such as weight bearing, prying). I call these three additional memory processes distribution, hyperassociation, and proceduralization. When I think about my own imaginary experiences while I am dreaming, these ideas take on a strong common-sense appeal.

Dreaming has several features that could enhance all four of these functions. For the function of memory consolidation, REM sleep provides a time when the brain-mind does not have to accept new data. It also provides an altered chemistry — a neuromodulation of the circuitry with the help of acetylcholine — that may permit the conversion of short-term memory into long-term memory. For the memory distribution function, REM sleep provides a massive, widespread activation with intense reiterative stimulation of all the cortical circuits of the brain. For the hyperassociation function, REM sleep provides the co-activation of newly sensitized circuits and all those circuits previously endowed with the multiple interconnections necessary for category overinclusiveness. For the proceduralization function, REM sleep provides the automatic running of motor programs that give the data access to existing action files.

In short, dream scenes are random and we impose a plot. In doing so, we are cementing memories and linking them to action programs. This is one major reason why we must sleep. One surprising implication of this theory is that the outward calm of sleep is entirely misleading. The motor programs in the brain are never more active than during REM sleep! As our dreams make clear, REM sleep entails a frenzy of action — we run, we drive, we fly, we swim. There is no rest in REM sleep for the central programs that move us about by day. On the contrary, they are souped up, and we assume for good reason: to prevent their decay from disuse, to rehearse for their future actions when called on during waking, and to embed themselves in a rich matrix of meaning.

We must therefore pay homage to behavorism and B. F. Skinner, even though this notion would make him turn over in his grave. I suggest that memory is organized within a framework of motor programs within the brain. Far from being a black box of no relevance to behavorist psychology, the brain is a jack-in-the-box, filled to the brim with spring-loaded plans of action. As such it is the very wellspring of all behavior. These brain-mind behavior programs, like sensory representations, are virtual — and they have even been called "fictive" to capture their promissory aspect — but they are no less real. In our being and in our becoming, they are us and we are they.

CONFABULATION IN WAKING, DREAMING, AND FANTASY

The brain-mind is a storyteller in all its states. After the alarm clock rings, it enters its nonfiction mode and says: "Time to get up. It's Wednesday. Don't forget to stop by the bank. You have a consultation downtown this morning. You have an appointment at 2:00 P.M. at the hospital. Your 5:00 P.M. seminar topic is Dreams and Fantasies. Remember to make a supper reservation at Ciao Bella."

This level of plot outlining is familiar to all of us. Every day we write out the sequence of scenarios that constitute the action programs for our lives. To do this we need access to recent memory, to remote memory, and to orientational data. And we need to be able to tie the plan to our motor programs and run them. This process is so routine that we tend to take it for granted.

The foreground level of narration is not the whole story, however. As soon as we get moving, perhaps even when we look in the mirror while still brushing our teeth, a parallel narrative kicks in. "You look tired today," you say to your image. Or you say, "You are irresistible when you smile." Like James Thurber's Walter Mitty, some of us can become so totally absorbed in these private fictions that we miss the change of the traffic lights. Until someone beeps!

The storylike strain of mental activity that proceeds in parallel with our minute-to-minute perceptions, thoughts, and actions has been called reflection, daydreaming, woolgathering, and fantasy (the term I prefer). For many people, fantasy is so much in the background that it is scarcely conscious at all. But if we pay a little attention, we can see that it occurs at some level all the time. The background fantasy process is so closely connected to the reality program in the foreground of consciousness that it often initiates rehearsals for upcoming social encounters. Fantasy also serves to review our recently completed interactions with others. We say to ourselves, "I wish I had said such and such" or "That went surprisingly well."

These little fictions also offer us the comfort of humorous self-reflection, as when we imagine ourselves as Woody Allen playing the brilliant fool or Albert Einstein playing the spontaneous genius. For erotic consolation we might become Henry Miller or Josephine Baker and play the compulsive lover, irresistible and insatiable. In this sense fantasy is our art world, our private theater with its endless opportunity to escape from the banality of the everyday into the exotic land of imagination and creativity.

Years ago, while I was in college, a friend of mine reported his extreme anxiety at having to carry steel supplies across the girders of skyscraper skeletons during a summer job he had in New York City. The pay was great, but the emotional cost was exorbitant. The worst of it, he said, was that he couldn't really talk to his fellow workers; he needed their support and comradeship to help him cope while passing rivets. One afternoon, on the very highest floor, and on its outer girder edge, he tried to engage a union welder in diverting small talk.

"Quiet!" demanded the pro. "I'm having a mental." "Mental" was the welder's word for fantasy.

Later, in the locker room at ground level, the welder explained. "I was right in the middle of a hot sex scene with my girlfriend," he said. "You don't like to be interrupted when you are making love, do you?"

What are we to make of this curious story? That we can avoid anxiety by escape fantasy? That the brain, unlike the dupe of a bad joke, can do more than one job at a time? Or that fantasy represents a continuous, ongoing stream of subconscious impulses that constitute our instructional programs or survival strategies?

In the psychoanalytic era, it was common to assume that blatant wish fulfillment of sexual desires in fantasies like those of the welder proved there was a deep link between fantasizing and dreaming. Dreaming was a breakthrough, made when the waking gatekeeper of our socially unacceptable urges was off duty. The source of both fantasy and dreams was the repressed unconscious. And many modern psychologists who have washed their hands of Freud still assume that fantasy and dreams are qualitatively similar, that they reflect the undifferentiated activation of networks whose connections code the data of our secret and forbidden fables.

If this were so, we would expect the reports of fantasies and dreams from the same individuals to be formally indistinguishable. And we would expect to see in both the same quantitative scores of such formal properties as orientational instability.

Here is a transcript of one of Delia's fantasy reports.

While driving to school after a frustrating and stressful day at work, I imagined that I go to talk to a professor about doing work for him in primate research in Africa. He is thrilled to have me, and I talk it over with my family who think it's a great opportunity. I'll be gone for a couple of months. I plan the shots and clothes I'll need. Next I see myself walking in the jungle trying to follow some orangutans. I think to myself that they are more unpredictable than gorillas and feel uneasy. I see myself at night writing in my note-book in a tent. I'm mad at myself because I'm worrying about being away from my family. I realize I don't feel free to go on such an adventure, which makes me determine that if I ever get such an opportunity I'll take it.

The fantasy certainly seems different from Delia's dreams in several ways. But how so, exactly? I decided to test whether the reports of fantasies and dreams from the same individuals could be distinguished and if so, what fundamental qualities were different. I appealed to another one of my classes, this one a collection of Harvard University psychology students. Although the test revealed a large area of overlap — indicating that dreams and fantasies do share many brain-mind state features — there were also marked differences, indicating that each brain-mind state is unique, with its own distinctive signature.

Dreams turned out to be about two and one-half times as "crowded" as fantasies. That is, there were many more characters in dreams. There were also more settings in dreams, and those settings were generally more richly detailed and more exotic. They were also more remote, less likely to reflect where the dreamer had been today or could go in a day's drive. When time was specified (and it usually wasn't) dreams also tended to be more displaced from "the present" than fantasies.

A quick comparison of Delia's fantasy with her long dream report — about being in the balloon above Paris — shows all these distinctions well. There is only one character in Delia's fantasy, her professor, who is a well-defined, real person in her life. In her dream, there are four, and one of them (the hotel clerk) is not well defined. Although the settings change in Delia's fantasy, they are commonplace and literal, not extraordinary (like flying in a balloon) or improbable (the Al-Aqsa Mosque in Paris). Delia's fantasy took place at a specific time, even linked to a calendar, while her dream scenes took place in some weird distortions of the distant past and the future.

Some of the differences in places, persons, and times could be due to the fact that while we think we are awake in dreams, in fantasy, we really are awake. This means that fantasy always has a door open to the here and now through which local places, characters, and even time references can easily pass. But in dreams the door to the here and now is slammed shut — along with our eyes and other sensory portals.

Dream characters are not only more numerous, they have less definite identities. Even the people the dreamer knows well — like Delia's father — have peculiar characteristics in dreams, but not in fantasies. One distinctly dreamlike feature of persons — their tendency to change into someone else — is *never* seen in fantasy. This identity switching in dreams has been called transmogrification. Now, I have no doubt that some of us could get up a fantasy and, by autosuggestion, induce a character switch or two, but it does not occur when subjects leave their brain-minds to their own devices.

What does all this have to do with memory and its bed partner, confabulation? It means that *both* processes are constrained by the brain-mind states in which they occur. We can confabulate when we are awake or when we are in a dream. But the fact that the product will be different implies that the production process is also quite different.

The line between our foreground problem-solving cognition and our background impulse stream of fantasy, while usually clear, can become uncomfortably fuzzy. In no case is the fuzziness more distressing than in psychosis. Here the distinction breaks down entirely. Exotic myth can replace conventional thinking.

That's what happened just before Bertal's mother brought him to The Psycho. A provocative television scenario took over Bertal's narration generator. The result was a psychotic fiction of classic Oedipal proportions.

Two nights before his admission to The Psycho, Bertal and his mother had watched a TV show about a woman having a baby. Over the next forty-eight hours Bertal became more and more preoccupied with birth and became convinced that his mother, who had recently gained weight, was going to have another child. When his mother decided to bring Bertal in, she told him to get into the car and that they were "just going for a ride." When they reached

The Psycho, which Bertal of course recognized since he had been there for a stay on two previous occasions, he nonetheless told the staff in the admissions room that he was there because his mother was pregnant and he couldn't deliver the baby. When he was asked to sign in, he signed his father's name, because, he said, his father "couldn't make it."

Just as frustration at work moved Delia to fantasize about primate research in Africa, the TV show launched Bertal into his mother-pregnancy psychosis. In both cases, a real stimulus was the trigger for a fictive and elaborate confabulation. And in their confabulations, both Delia and Bertal focused on relationships with opposite-sex parental figures. In Delia's case, the imagery is more realizable than in Bertal's, and this reliability measures the difference between fantasy and psychosis. Furthermore, although both Delia's fantasy and Bertal's psychosis are dreamlike, they are clearly differentiated from dreaming in that they have highly focused, persistent themes involving relatively few, realistic characters. This suggests that a major difference between dreaming and fantasy or psychosis is the versatility of the confabulation.

DREAM SPLICING

One of the most precious myths about dreams — and one that I myself was always sure was true — is that, in spite of their microscopic chaos, their overall plot design is unified. It has even been maintained that the succession of dreams during a single night is like the chapters of a book. That is a very flattering concept: inside our heads is a little scenario writer who is so uncannily organized he can keep the big picture clear even when the individual images are fuzzy!

I was so convinced of this high-level dream-plot coherence that I was extolling what I took to be an indubitable example of it at a seminar. Although the dreamer jumped around from place to place and even from one continent to another in the dream report I was discussing, the whole dream seemed to me to be tightly held together by the continuing twine of familial relationship. The settings, characters, and actions were wildly disparate, but the dream seemed to be telling the story of the dreamer's life. So having dazzled myself and the group with what I called my "frame sequence method" (now in the ash bin), I said, "Despite the gibberish you can see that it all hangs together. It's a story."

"How can you be so sure?" asked my co-worker Bob Stickgold. "I'm not convinced at all." Having slept on the question himself for a few nights, Bob had come up with a very simple but heretofore unimagined experimental approach to test for cohesiveness. He called it dream splicing. Here is how we used it.

We took twenty random dream reports from twenty people, each of which were of about equal length and each of which contained one scene shift. We cut ten of the reports in half with a pair of scissors at the point where the scene shifted. That left us with ten dream heads and ten dream tails. We then transposed these pieces: heads on tails, heads on heads, tails on heads, tails on tails.

We then gave the ten spliced dreams and the ten unspliced dreams to members of the seminar and asked them to distinguish which reports were spliced crossovers and which were not. If dreams are telling stories and each dreamer has a particular story to tell, it ought to be easy on any one of a number of grounds to say, "Yes, that one is an intact story" and "No, that one surely is spliced!"

That night I sat down myself with my own set of reports and tried to sort them out. By the time I got to the third report, I had spent over thirty minutes in obsessive agony and all I had to show for it was a splitting headache, so I put the task aside for a while. Humiliation, shame, and guilt goaded me. I spent three more hours on the task and kept changing my judgments back and forth. My efforts were to no avail. I could not tell a spliced dream from an intact one. And no one in the group did much better than chance.

The significance of this is that, although each subplot may be a storylike unit, there is no story line connecting one subplot to the next. Dream coherence may be in the eye of the beholder, but it is *not* in the text of the reports. There is dramatic segmentation within dreams. Each story is gotten up under local constraints. The brain is jumping around. When we are awake we can concentrate on a subject for hours, but when we are asleep we can't focus for more than a few minutes. Freud thought, and others still maintain, that the dreams we have over the course of an entire night are integral. It cannot be. The evidence simply does not substantiate it.

WHOSE DREAMS ARE YOU DREAMING?

Are our dreams the same as those of everyone else? I believe that the dream-splicing evidence forces us to consider the possibility that they are, that the formal aspects of dreaming result from a change in brain-mind state that is universal, impersonal, and imperative.

While much more investigation remains to be done, it would appear that our dream amnesia and our dream confabulations are the impersonal necessities of a brain state that is forced on us by our nature. We can romanticize about dreams, tell ourselves we are receiving messages from the gods, or believe that some secret code is being broken to unveil an essential truth whose revelation will change our lives. But I honestly think that in entertaining such conceits we are being had by the dream romancers even more flagrantly than we are being had by the dreams themselves. At least the dream is free. The dream romancers charge us money for their code-breaking services.

In any case, it would appear that we are all easily fooled into thinking that dreams are intact stories when they are not. This seems to mean that one of the main predispositions of the integrated brain-mind is to discern integrity, unity, and singleness of purpose in any text that appears to be integral. And when integrity does not reside in the text, we impute it. This recognition renders not just dream interpretation, but the whole interpretative exercise of humanistic criticism and scholarship, extremely problematic.

Now we can see, even more clearly, why Freud and Jung were both right and wrong when they said, "Let the dreamer awake and you will see psychosis." Yes, Delia's dreams and fantasies and Bertal's psychosis are all alike in that they are confabulatory. But the dreaming confabulation is so lush and lavish it is distinctly different from the other two states. Only in a flagrant organic psychosis, like the DTs of alcohol withdrawal, does confabulation assume truly dreamlike proportions. This must mean that fantasy, dreaming, and psychosis are on the same continuum of states but that each state on the continuum has its own distinctive character reflecting its own specific brain activation pattern.

CHAPTER 8

Seeing Is Believing: Perception and Hallucination

CAN'T BELIEVE MY EYES" is an expression we often use when we witness an unusual event. I said it just the other day when I was standing on the terrace of a condominium and I saw a flock of goats walking along the sandy beach before me. It was like a scene from a Buñuel movie — there was even a scraggly-looking shepherd with a crook, a cloak, and an energetic mutt to keep the flock in order. But this was not a film. What was the explanation for goats on the beach? I must have been out of my mind.

Turns out the explanation was simple. The town to which I had repaired to think and write part of this book was in Sicily, where the agrarian past and the urban present are seamlessly merged. The spatial incongruity of goats in front of a condo on the beach was normal in view of the local socioeconomic situation.

Because I was an outsider, I was the only one who was surprised by the goat parade. The native passerby whom I questioned about it calmly explained that the goats were simply on their way to the high mountain pastures that surround Taormina.

The fact is, we have to believe our eyes. It's our only hope. If we went around thinking our vision was suspect, we would drown in a sea of self-doubt. Most of the time, we are right to believe our eyes. I mean, there really were goats on that beach.

But how can we be sure that it is our eyes that are doing the seeing? The answer is already clear from our dream experience: we can't. The visual system of our brain-mind is completely capable of simulating the world with such skill that it fools us every time we go to sleep and dream. It fools me. And Delia. And Bertal. All that is needed to get us into big trouble is a shift in the balance between external stimuli and internal stimuli. This is because vision actually takes place within the brain-mind. Our conviction that what we see is "out there" is a deep delusion.

The images we "see" are only representations of the real world. When we point our heads at a tree, our eyes receive light waves that are bouncing off that tree. The light input is computed by our brains, the computation is checked against data stored in our neurons, and the resulting match tells us the light signals we have received constitute a tree. To a fly with its compound eyes, the same light signals produce a very different picture. By now we've all seen those infrared images of a house or a person's body that show with computer-enhanced color which areas are hot and which are cool. The objects produce the same light waves, but the receiver, in this case an instrument, "sees" the data differently.

Hearing also works this way. Think about the dog whistle, which emits a very high pitch. We can't hear it, but Fido comes running. Why can't we hear it? After all, the sound waves hitting our eardrums are the same ones as those hitting Fido's. But his brain can process them, and ours can't.

Seeing and hearing are perceptions. Our eyes and ears survey the world, constantly, to let us know what's going on. Considering that we do not perceive anything directly, but only after our brain has processed the incoming signal, it would seem that we are on the razor's edge of madness all the time. Why is the brain-mind designed in such a risky way? How is the delicate balance maintained? Could the changes in brain-mind states between waking and dreaming actually serve to protect us from madness? And can the brain-mind state theory help explain how we perceive and how our perceptions can go wrong? Let's try to answer some of these questions.

HOW WE SEE

In order for the eye to see it must be moving. In fact, the eyes are in motion even when we fix them on an object of interest. Sounds incredible, doesn't it? You can't feel the movement. You can't even see it; try it, by looking into a mirror, or the eyes of a loved one. And so you tend to doubt this whole story. But the evidence is overwhelming.

Even when the object you are looking at is motionless, your eyes move imperceptibly all the time. Scientists who study vision in the lab use eye-tracking machines that can gauge the movements. It is the eyeball itself that moves, in tiny, fast, flicking motions. Part of the reason you can't see it is because the brain cancels out tiny movements in all the images you perceive, in order to keep them from jumping or blurring, just as the tracking-control button on your VCR keeps the video image from flickering. If the eye muscles are paralyzed, vision ceases. No eye movement, no vision.

The converse is also true. When scientists shine light on the retina and record the electrical signals sent into the brain, they find they can excite the retinal neurons only by moving or flashing the light source. The cells of the retina are interested only in changes in the properties of the light, not in the fixed properties.

Paralyzing the eye muscles is not the only way to impair vision. The brain-stem nerve cells that command the eyes can be damaged so that certain eye movements become impossible. The astonishing fact is that when a person who has been injured in this way tries, unsuccessfully, to move the eyes, the world itself seems to flicker. The reason for this illusion is that when the brain stem sends motor commands to the eye muscles, it sends simultaneous messages to the visual-processing regions of the cortex, to help it predict the changing scene to come. The brain-mind uses these signals to prevent the visual image from blurring or jumping while the eyes are actually moving. The visual brain-mind is constantly adjusting its own image by converting movement commands from the brain stem into sensory position data in the cortex. So the brain-mind of the injured person is making adjustments for eye movement, but there is no actual eye movement going on. The result is an internally generated flicker.

Since eye movements can be recorded in waking as well as sleep, the test for this theory is simply to attach electrodes to the skin around a person's eyes and ask him to fix upon a stationary target and follow it when it moves. Electrical recordings in waking subjects reveal that the eyes make upward of twenty small, rapid movements per second. Animal experiments show that this constant agitation is highly organized with many, many brain-stem cells contributing to its administration. Even though they are small, the micromovements result in a significant and constant change in the properties of light falling on the retina of each eye, enabling the brain to process images.

Thus vision is a double illusion: the world is stable, but I can't see it unless my eyes move, yet by moving my eyes, I make the images jump, which my brain then corrects again so that the final illusion is stable!

If you are still in any doubt whatsoever, think about this one. If I were to hook you up to an eye-movement recorder and display your eye position as a dot of light on a screen across the room, such that each eye movement you made caused the dot to move, what do you think you would see? A dot moving around the screen is the obvious answer. But you won't see the dot move at all. All you will see is a sequence of stationary dots. Everyone else in the room will see the dots actually move from one position to another. This effect is called "visual blanking," implying that during the eye movements, vision is actually suppressed.

One way to appreciate this process is to recognize how a movie reel works. There is a black band separating each frame of the movie, but if the projector moves the reel at faster than twelve frames a second, your eyes will not perceive the black line as it zips up across the screen; it goes by too fast. This is a result of visual blanking; you believe that the movement of the objects depicted on the screen is continuous rather than intermittent. The black bar that you see hovering on your television screen when the vertical control is not set properly is the result of the same phenomenon; in fact, engineers call it the vertical blanking interval.

SLEEP DEPRIVATION AND HALLUCINATION

Once we appreciate the fact that our "normal" vision is a reproduction of reality, it should be easier for us to understand how the brain-mind creates entirely artificial visions. As we will see, we can shift our brain-mind states voluntarily to improve our health; in the same way, shifts can be made in the interests of having a religious experience — if we want to have a vision, there is an easy way.

Visions, hallucinations, dreams — call them what you will — are all actively invited by seekers of spiritual truth. The perceptions are often achieved by entering an uncommon state, be it trance, meditation, or other ritual practice. A very curious and informative case is that of Emanuel Swedenborg, the seventeenth-century Swedish botanist turned evangelist. On the basis of his visions, he created the Church of the New Jerusalem, a branch of Protestant religion. He used a particularly interesting technique for inducing the visions that informed his religious doctrines: sleep deprivation.

Swedenborg worked in an era when "science" simply meant knowledge, all knowledge, and a scientist was measured as much by the breadth as by the depth of his intellect. Swedenborg's knowledge was so broad that he wrote treatises on botany, zoology, geology, and astronomy. He also was sure that science would ultimately lead him to a direct encounter with God. But the heavenly Father failed to appear in the lenses of his microscopes or telescopes.

Disappointed but undaunted, Swedenborg set out to sharpen his powers of internal observation, his insight, if you will. Resuscitating the medievalists' use of dreams as a vehicle of revelation, he systematically undertook a program of dream sensitization and dream enhancement. His method is classical and effective; I have learned to use it in my own self-experiments. Whether one is bent on an as-yet-unfulfilled career as a charismatic or simply interested to see if dreams are as frequent and long as scientists say they are, it is possible for anyone to repeat Swedenborg's procedures.

The rules are simple: (1) keep a dream journal, (2) keep irregular hours, (3) get up before you have satiated your need for sleep. That's all there is to it.

As Swedenborg discovered, by paying attention to dreams he noticed them more, and by writing them down in his journal, he paid more attention to them. This in turn caused him to notice dreams even more. And so on. The journal is all you really need. But if you throw in irregular hours, you will increase your yield appreciably because you will have a much greater tendency to wake up at unexpected times, thereby increasing your chances of waking up just after, or even during, a dream.

I have said nothing about the content of the ambushed dreams. And indeed it doesn't matter. If you want religious visions, you can probably induce them. If you want Freudian or Jungian dreams, you can induce them too. Dream content is heavily context dependent, which is why we ignore it in scientific endeavors and concentrate on dream form. Dream form is universal, so we feel justified in assuming that it faithfully reflects brain activity.

So far we have talked only about increasing the frequency of recalling your dreams. But if you add sleep deprivation you can also increase the intensity of your dreams, as Swedenborg knew and every other visionary wanna-be has discovered. Our drive to dream is like other instincts such as hunger, thirst, and sex. Stop doing any of these things for a while and your appetite increases, and so does your satisfaction when you are finally fulfilled. Swedenborg found that by keeping himself awake all night and then letting himself sleep fitfully by day his dreams were more intense. For him, that meant that God appeared more often and with more cogent and urgent instructions about what needed to be done to properly reform the religious theory and practice of the day.

MY RED-EYE VISION

Our need to dream, or, I should say, to perceive internally generated stimuli, is a stronger drive than we might want to believe. I learned that for myself one day some years ago. I had been at a busy scientific meeting in Anaheim, California, for five days, and I was to fly back to Boston on one of those well-named red-eye flights. On this particular flight I got even less sleep than usual because I was seated next to an intriguing female colleague; our conversation was so scintillating we didn't sleep a wink.

The dawn over Lake Erie was glorious, and we landed in Boston in the middle of one of those high-pressure weather systems that makes the New England fall so exhilarating. High and dry with a blue, blue sky. At the airport I was met by my family for our not-to-be-missed annual outing in Vermont. Knowing my sleepless state, I did not drive, but tried to nap in the back of our station wagon. Aroused by the road's bumps, my kids' jumps, and my encounter in the airplane, I didn't succeed.

Having arrived at my farm, I wanted to begin to get my winter wood in order. We would probably need a fire that night. And the day was so gloriously clear that I decided to forgo sleep and get the chores done. I felt fine. Even a bit elated. I was not tired. Not groggy. Not dreamy or even daydreamy. I was lucid and energetic. Sharp.

After a quick lunch (at about 8:00 A.M. Anaheim time) I was stacking kindling in neat piles under the tin roof of my lean-to woodshed. It is somewhat dark under the roof, but there was still plenty of light to see by. Suddenly, I had an unexpected helper. He was standing behind my right shoulder. At first, I couldn't really see him, but I could definitely sense his presence. When I turned my head and eyes to the light, sure enough, there he was. The only problem was that I hadn't hired a helper. And Vermonters, as friendly as they are, don't usually just turn up like that, especially total strangers; and this guy was utterly unknown to me. My heart started pounding like a log splitter and I was overcome with terror.

Though I must have run from the shed I only remember reeling with vertigo, nausea, and panic as I spun and fell to the ground about fifteen feet from where I had seen him. When I stood up in the clear, cool air I was relieved to discover that there wasn't really anyone else by the woodshed after all. After I regained my composure I went back to sorting kindling and got the job done before recounting my adventure to my family over dinner.

My son Chris wanted to know how long the strange episode

had lasted. I guessed about two seconds, certainly no more than five. When he asked me what I thought had happened, all I could say was that I had a visual hallucination accompanied by intense panic and anxiety. It was hard in retrospect to say which came first, the vision or the fear. I guessed that they were simultaneous. At first both elements were quite mild, but they seemed to grow, together; it was like a nightmare and a seizure all rolled into one. There was a strange aura at the beginning — the vague sense of a presence. I turned to look and then I saw him. I felt scared and then I lost consciousness for an instant. Then I reeled, spun, and fell as if driven down to the ground.

I'm happy to report it's the only frank hallucination I have ever had and that my EEG is normal. I have had no seizures before or since. Some people think I'm a bit eccentric, maybe bizarre, but not even my severest critics use the word "psychotic." So how do we explain this?

One answer springs immediately to mind. The deprivation of sleep that I incurred during my red-eye flight from Los Angeles to Boston caused my brain to be hyperexcitable. Vision neurons that would normally respond only to external stimuli were now prone to fire impulsively on their own, as if they had lost an important restraining force.

Recall that when we are awake the amines keep acetylcholine in check. When we are in REM sleep, the amines can no longer restrain the acetylcholine molecules, which trigger the hallucinations we see as dreams. Could it be that by resting in REM sleep the amines are better able to do their restraining job on acetylcholine during the next day? And could it be, then, that since my amines had not had a rest of their own, they finally crumbled under the excessive pressure of acetylcholine while I was standing at the woodshed? We must take these ideas seriously because they promise not only to explain the deleterious effects of sleep deprivation but to tell us about the beneficial effects of sleep itself.

Putting Swedenborg's story and mine together suggests a theory: that the balance of our internal electrical excitation and inhibition is so finely tuned that the brain-mind is always on the edge of seizurelike hallucinations. In this theory, the job of sleep is to protect or stabilize that balance, so that perception can be creative enough to reproduce the world but not so creative that it produces entirely artificial worlds. What would happen to us, then, if we were to suddenly and violently shift the balance in favor of electrical excitation?

DREAMS AS SEIZURE

I have always been astonished — and horrified — by the crudeness of electroshock treatment. Basically, the brain-mind is plugged into the Edison company. The electric current causes such a massive overdrive of the brain cells that a seizure is triggered. This is followed by a period of unconsciousness. When I was in training to be a psychiatrist, I found shock therapy to be morally and intellectually unacceptable because it was not only crude but inexplicable. To reduce the chance of injury that the intense muscle contractions associated with the seizure might cause, patients who are to undergo shock treatment are given a curare-like drug that partially paralyzes their muscles, adding the risk of respiratory arrest to an already frightening procedure.

You can thus imagine my amazement and consternation when a depressed man came into The Psycho's outpatient clinic one day and demanded electroshock therapy. I advised him that we had drugs that were much safer and every bit as effective in treating depressions. But the fact is, shock therapy is often dramatically effective, and this particular patient had tried both therapies and found that the shock treatments were not only quicker, but enabled him to avoid the side effects he got from the drugs. He claimed that three or four shocks were all that he needed to avert the horrible sinking hole of depression that he was falling into. He was afraid that his depression would last six months if we didn't act fast.

I checked out his chart, consulted widely, and then did as he had asked. And as he had predicted, his mood bounced right back. I will spare you a description of the seizures he underwent, which still haunt my memory. At the time, I hadn't heard of REM sleep, but I recall wondering how and why such a massive overdriving of the brain could have such prompt and lasting effects on a person's mood.

My theory now is that the artificially induced state of brain-mind hyperexcitability, in which the motor output is blocked by a drug, is something like REM sleep, and that it's possible to look at REM sleep as a modified seizure. In other words, my theory is homeopathic: we have a sleep seizure in order to avoid a waking seizure. We dream so as not to hallucinate.

If you were to look at the EEG of a patient during a seizure, you would see that the ominously spiked traces that are diagnostic of epilepsy look just like the PGO waves in REM sleep. The difference is in the source; in an epileptic fit, the source of the waves is usually high up in the cortex, but during REM sleep the source is deep down in the base of the brain stem. As we know, that is the center of state control — it's the battleground for the aminergic-cholinergic system.

The PGO waves represent unbridled brain-cell electricity. "Brain-stem lightning bolts" is hyperbolic but to the point. They spread like flash fire to areas of the brain, exciting them wildly. The electrical fire of REM sleep flashes in the same way, upward to the visual brain (which sees), sideways to the movement and balance system (which flicks the eyes), and down to body-movement command cells.

A look at the EEG indicates that the dreamy states of epileptics may not be all that different from those we experience during dreaming. And the modified seizures that we induce by electroshock may not be all that different from the physiological experience we have during dreams. Furthermore, the ease of experimentally inducing a seizure is increased when the subject has had sleep deprivation. Sleep has the effect of restoring the usual protection against seizures that most of us enjoy all of our lives. There is also reason to believe that REM sleep offers insurance of another kind — it may help prevent psychosis, a state which, we are learning, may depend in part on a shift in the balance of excitation within the brain.

If this theory is correct, there ought to arise — as a cruel experiment of nature — cases in which REM sleep's capacity to prevent natural seizures is missing. During REM sleep the brain stem blocks the motor commands, so certain damage to the brain stem ought to negate this action, allowing those commands to reach muscles during a dream scenario. It now seems this may be so; recently, scientists have uncovered cases in which dreams are acted out owing to a failure in inhibition of motor commands.

THE MAN WHO MISTOOK HIS WIFE FOR A BEND IN THE ROAD

José was sixty-three years old when he and his wife, Giovanna, came to see me in the early 1980s about their sleep problem. I asked them both to keep records of what happened. Here are two of José's journal entries:

> 1. I was dreaming. I was in the midst of driving on an extreme curve to the left. I tried to maneuver. My wife woke me up — I had hit her on the arm (not hard) with my elbow.
> 2. I was dreaming. This guy used to be a football star quarterback. They're having him do this movie stunt. I don't know what he had to do, but there was this big sphere (way up in the sky). I was up there too and the metal object was spinning. It was coming at me and I was ducking. When my wife awakened me, I was sitting up in bed holding my arms up thinking, If this hits me, it's all over.

Many years earlier it had been clearly shown that sleepwalking occurs in non-REM sleep and is *not* associated with dreaming. People who sleepwalk are not acting out a dream. During non-REM sleep, motor activity is not blocked, so our bodies are free to move about. We rarely do more than roll over in bed, though, because there is little brain activity during non-REM periods (sleepwalking is discussed further in chapter 14). The occasional reports from patients and their bed partners of dramatic and often fearsome dream enactments were therefore perplexing, because we brain-mind scientists had assumed that the inhibition of motor output in REM sleep was almost always effective. Our assumptions overlooked two points. First, even strong inhibition is only relative; although the spinal nerves that normally command movement are dampened, they can be turned on if the excitation is strong enough. The other point is that the degree of inhibition may vary from time to time and person to person, especially if the inhibitory nerves in the brain stem are lost due to disease or aging.

In retrospect, it's pretty obvious that José was having visuomotor hallucinations of the sort that are typical of dreams and that he was actually moving exactly as he imagined himself to be moving in the dream. It is also obvious from the examples above and others in his journal that the dreams in which movement actually broke through the inhibitory barrier were those in which he felt a strong sense of threat or danger. José was trying to avert disaster on the hairpin curve (but in doing so whacked his wife); next, he was desperately trying to avoid a spinning metal object coming toward him (and found himself stretching out his arms in self-defense). Other dreams drove him right out of bed, face first on the floor, causing significant pain and injury.

We knew from Giovanna's notes and tape recordings that José's dream enactments were occurring in REM sleep, because she could see that eye movements and facial grimaces usually preceded the thrashing and twisting of José's trunk and limbs, which she said were "like he was having a fit." Sleep lab recordings of patients like José have now confirmed that, indeed, the dreamed motor acts are somehow breaking through the normally protective barrier of inhibition. We can liken REM-sleep motor inhibition to the clutch in an automobile. During inhibition the clutch is disengaged; the engine is humming along but no power reaches the wheels. Were it not for this physiological clutch, all our dream motors would be connected to our wheels and we would be thrashing about every night of our lives!

We're lucky. And so was José, whose worst fear was actually hurting his wife, Giovanna, whom he deeply loved. That never happened. Because she was a light sleeper, Giovanna was able to dodge José's dream-driven flailing and awaken him to stop the process. Having successfully defeated an alcohol problem earlier in his life, José was reluctant to take the medication that was newly available — and effective — in treating his condition, which is called REM sleep behavior disorder. As is so often the case, José was helped most by having three strong pillars of natural support: increased understanding of the nature of the problem, acceptance of the problem as a variation on a normal process, and a significant degree of control over his sleep that he achieved with meditation and relaxation. Just as José had earlier recognized the need to stop drinking, he now recognized the need to give up his late nights, his high-strung lifestyle, and his irregular sleep schedule.

MOTOR-PATTERN GENERATORS

What causes REM sleep behavior disorder? Can it be cured or just symptomatically relieved? It is still too early to know. In all likelihood this unusual brain-mind state has different causes. Any process that affects the brain-stem motor inhibitory center, or the pathways from it to the muscles, could weaken the restraint on unwarranted movement. And any process that overdrives the motor-pattern generators of the brain stem and thus increases the excitation of movement neurons in the spinal cord could cause the disorder.

This disorder is among the strongest evidence that dreams are linked, and even driven, by motor programs in the brain stem. When he's awake, José's visual world, like all of ours, is driven by motor inputs — the tiny motions of our eyes. When he's dreaming, however, José's clutch sometimes does not disengage, and the motor in his brain, idling away at top speed, runs his dream around the bedroom!

Bertal also had a problem with his motor programs. His episodes of strong hallucination often made him catatonic. His posture became rigid and he assumed bizarre statuesque poses. There was something wrong with his motor system, just as there was with his visual excitation. After one episode at The Psycho, I found Bertal squatting in the kitchen staring at the wall. I spoke to him for an hour while he remained motionless, tucked in an awkward ball. He gave no reply, except for one instant when he asked, "Why do I do the foolish things I do?"

Bertal's motor and visual systems also were out of kilter when my supervisor had entered the seclusion room where the orderlies had put Bertal after one of his terrifying war hallucinations. Bertal first mistook him as the "enemy," then began flailing away at him.

The evidence from both José and Bertal seems to indicate clearly that bizarre movement and bizarre perceptions are linked in many altered brain-mind states. The sensory system doesn't work properly when the motor-system programs are running afoul, and vice versa. The brain-mind is a unified system and, for better or worse, it is unified by its states.

When we decide we want to go somewhere, we voluntarily initiate movement sequences. Once they begin, though, the sequences are so automatic that they no longer require our conscious supervision. Walking, jogging, even sprinting are gaits controlled by brain-stem motor-pattern generators. All we have to do is flip a command switch in our cortex and our lower brain coordinates the motion. Because that command center is in the cortex, and the centers for gait control are in the brain stem and spinal cord, our decision to walk is one of many examples of what scientists call a top-down process.

There are situations in which it is advantageous to short-circuit the cortex and activate a motor-pattern generator directly from the brain stem. If we suddenly see a car careening toward us, we instantly turn our car away; we react automatically, and only later (even if it is only a split second later) do we realize there is danger and feel afraid. The startle response and the orienting response are also good examples of short-circuit processes. Because in these cases the brain-stem signals precede thought, they are called bottom-up processes.

Whether or not the motor-pattern generators are under voluntary (top-down) or automatic (bottom-up) control depends on our state. The gait control circuits are in the brain stem, intertwined with the same networks that govern brain-mind states. We can see this in the lab — we can stimulate and change the gait control circuits in the brain stem electrically or with chemicals.

We can also see this anecdotally. José's effort to correct the course of his dream car was a voluntary effort to regain control.

It was top-down. It interrupted the normal bottom-up process of dreaming, which inhibits motor output. We certainly feel we are making voluntary motions when we are in fear in our own dreams. We try to run from imaginary assailants, and we too would feel we were throwing our arms up in self-defense if we were to suddenly turn around in a dream and see a huge metal sphere screaming toward our heads. In such perilous moments we actually will ourselves to run away, to block the sphere. It is then that the REM-sleep dream state is most likely to break. These top-down movement commands from the cortex override the signals from the brain stem; they break through the motor inhibition, and we wake up, often in terror, and in a cold sweat.

THE PRIMACY OF MOVEMENT

Why do such motor programs run in our sleep, and aren't there some dangers in their doing so? What if the boundaries become blurred? What really stops José from assaulting his wife if he supposes she is an intruder? And what does all this have to do with the relationship between brain-mind states and the faculty of perception? By the end of this chapter, I hope to offer some answers.

To this point, I have discussed how external and internal vision work and how vision is integrated with movement, and indeed how movement itself is an active organizer of sensory experience. A look at how we develop in our early embryonic life will lead us to an even deeper proposition — that motor patterns are elemental building blocks of the brain. I will suggest that innate motor programs are functional blueprints for behaviors that are run by our brains in utero. The human fetus spends most of its last uterine days in a REM-like state that long antedates the emergence of conscious experience.

The question of "which comes first, brain or mind?" is a variation on the theme "which comes first, the chicken or the egg?" Speaking developmentally, most neuroscientists would say that the brain precedes the mind. The developing brain is dynamic, and there is an ordered movement at every level, from the rolling of the DNA printing press to the ceaseless flux of activity of cell membranes; from the serpentine twists of the embryo to the agitated dance of the fetus on the sonar screens of obstetrical offices around the world. We are forced by the evidence to consider motor acts as primary and formative as well as secondary and reactive.

All of life is flux. All of life is motion. Motion is perpetual. Broadening the definition of behavior to include even the microscopic movements that occur continuously within all living cells makes it clear that a very early organizational state of our existence is like REM sleep. Our primordial selves are twitching, writhing, and moving, and our eyes are wandering, in a uterine hot tub. No one can deny that this is motor behavior. Whether there is any psychology at these early stages is a matter of heavy moral weight that we cannot assess at this stage of our knowledge. But even if there is some primordial conscious experience — such as sensory processing that could be felt at some level — there is certainly no evidence whatsoever that we have the self-reflective awareness that is the essence of what we imply by the term consciousness.

We can avoid the philosophical quicksand of trying to decide precisely when consciousness begins by saying simply that we all spent a very significant amount of time in a very REM-like state before we were born. With new technology, embryologists can see eye movements in fetuses only twenty weeks old. And the earlier a premature baby is born, the more time it spends in REM sleep. That state, with or without consciousness, is characterized by automatic activation and motility. This set of observations has led many researchers to propose that REM sleep is a functional blueprint for human behavior. On the drawing boards of the womb, brain circuits are laid out and tested by an automatic process that probably arises as soon as the networks of nerve cells are first formed. Primordial movement is a building block of behavior. It helps the brain and the central nervous system complete and correct its wiring.

This is a classic example of self-organization, that amazing property of all complex systems to create order out of chaos. Our brains are programmed by periodic activation that begins in utero and resumes every night of our lives. And once we have set the brain-mind in motion, all we have to do is shape and modify it by experience. This is what it means to learn. We thus build what we have learned into the dynamic structure of an automatically active system. At some point early in life, the system acquires a rich enough stock of images and thoughts to have conscious awareness. Add a few more and it has enough to be aware that it is aware. Once we have self-reflective awareness, we are fully conscious.

In sketching this developmental model, several important new concepts have surfaced that will require continued attention. To the notion that brain-mind states are organizational units of enormous importance, we have added the idea that elemental building blocks of such states are motor patterns. In REM sleep, the automatic activation of motor patterns gets a self-organizing process going that gives the system the capacity for continuous and progressive change. That change is what we call maturation.

Now we can add still another new concept — that of procedural knowledge. Given that the fetus knows how to enter a REM-like state, it already possesses procedural knowledge. The fetus can't give an account of how it does this because it doesn't yet have narrative or implicit knowledge — but it does know how to do it.

Even later, when we are fully mature, most of our knowledge is procedural. We know how to tie our shoes. And we probably could write a five- or six-page paper explaining exactly how. But it is infinitely simpler to demonstrate the behavior. That is why we would rather show someone how to tie his shoes than to try to describe how to do it.

When it comes to swallowing, we don't even consider demonstrating how to do it. We just do it. This important behavior is completely self-taught, completely unconscious, and completely procedural. We can't remember learning to swallow because no one ever taught us to do it. We always knew how to swallow, long before the time of our earliest memory, long before, indeed, we were born. When fetuses suck their thumbs they may be fine-tuning the crucial act of swallowing.

MOVEMENT IS THE KEY TO LEARNING

For babies to survive in the world, they need to be born knowing how to do certain things. Because it is so crucial to feeding, swallowing is clearly one of them. This example shows that instincts are more or less collections of procedures. The technical term for such automatically programmed behaviors is "fixed acts." If we extended the list from feeding to, say, sex, we would again agree that many elements of even that behavior are present at birth. The erection of the phallus is one such behavior that begins in the womb and occurs during REM sleep for life.

When did you, as a baby, emit your first smile? Do you remember those baby pictures of you grinning, giving your mother evidence that she was doing her job effectively? Chances are that neither the camera nor your mother's eye caught your first smile because it might well have occurred before you were born. And it certainly did occur, often, when you were REMing away in your bassinet, unseen by any member of your loving family.

Smiles of happiness, frowns of displeasure, and grimaces of pain are among the many motor acts that have a truly instinctual character. As any parent of a demanding infant can attest, babies are born with an impressive repertoire of emotional displays, including that sleep-shattering scream that calls for feedings twice a night. These behaviors are preprogrammed by the self-activated brain, in REM, long before they are put to the service of survival.

Now that we recognize this self-organizing capacity of the brain-mind and its states, our whole concept of what Freud called infantile sexuality can change. We no longer need to endow such acts with intention or to project adult ideas of sexuality upon the newborn. We can abandon this forced explanation now that we understand the programmed automaticity of brain-mind states that extends into so many aspects of our mental life.

This change in viewpoint does not imply that sex is any less important, nor does it ignore the fact that sexual behavior can be messed up by societal pressures and prohibitions. The self-organization concept merely relegates sex to one of an equally important number of procedures that is actively and automatically developed over many years so that we, as babies, can be successful as human beings. Knowing about self-organization, we can now confidently say to parents, "Look, your job is much easier than you supposed because so much of the sculpting of all socially critical behavior is internal. You don't have to teach your child most procedural knowledge. In time, it will emerge spontaneously and naturally, especially if left to its own devices."

The purpose of laying such heavy emphasis on the motor side of the development story is to prepare the way for the idea that procedures may well be the nuclei for much of what seems to be purely sensory (as in my woodpile hallucination) or purely cognitive (as in Bertal's delusion about why he was coming to The Psycho). Every sensory experience, be it veridical or illusory, involves both action and belief, both movement and concept. In the case of vision, the crucial and fundamental role of eye movement is clear. Eye movement is likewise central to the orienting response. And, as such, it interacts with orientation, that vital faculty that we examined earlier. Through motion, we train our brain.

WE DREAM SO THAT WE MAY LEARN

When we find ourselves in a new place, we at once begin to develop orientational schemas. We build up our brain-mind maps by incorporating the results of exploring the environment and moving through it, while at the same time sniffing it, hearing it, and feeling its textures. This leads us to an important question that is tougher than it looks: How can we most efficiently and effectively assure that the orientational experience we perceive gets built into our system? In addition, how can we be sure that if a built-in procedure isn't used, it doesn't get lost?

One way would be to have a state (waking) in which we are exposed to new information and another state (REM sleep) in which the new data is integrated with the whole set of existing programs in the system. For that to happen, we would need to run the system automatically for a considerable length of time each day (say one and a half hours, the usual grand total of REM sleep for a night); we would want to run it fast (say six procedures a second, the usual rate of PGO wave signals); we would want to run it with the clutch disengaged (so the system does not have to output); and we would want to run it in an altered chemical climate (to favor a set of molecular operations that differs from that in waking, to encode long-term memory). That's a tall order. But it's all done reliably, efficiently, and unconsciously in REM sleep, the mother of all procedures! We are performing mental gymnastics, using motor programs to train our brain each time we dream.

That this process does not always occur perfectly we have already seen. Parts of it can get out of control. If we don't get enough sleep, visuomotor hallucinations may break through right into the light of day, as they did for me at the woodshed. If there are even small shifts of balance in the aminergic-cholinergic control system, motor acts may break through the inhibition of REM sleep, as they did for José. And if there are even more massive shifts in our sensorimotor modulators, we might all see dive-bombers and curl up in a tight ball as Bertal did that day at The Psycho.

We can even imagine some behaviors that have the properties of both REM sleep and seizure-driven fugues, in which elaborate violent acts could occur. In fact, the courts have recently considered several cases of nocturnal murder, in which the perpetrators willingly confessed and convinced juries of their peers that their acts were automatic and involuntary.

These startling dream enactments only emphasize what we already know if we have paid even passing attention to our own dreams. They are so full of imaginings — from thieves breaking into hotels, to flying high in a balloon over Paris, to veering off a sharp curve — that REM sleep must be preparing and equipping us for almost any possible waking eventuality. The programs are all there. Life's events call them forth. And, most of the time, they otherwise stay put.

We have our well-tempered sequence of brain-mind states to thank for that. The lessons of this chapter teach us that in order to see, we need to recreate the visual world in our brain-mind. This deeply artistic act requires that we scan the world by the perceptual jitter of our eyeballs, which means that our visions, be they veridi-

cal or fanciful, are all tightly tied to brain-stem motor-pattern generators. No wonder, then, that these motor mainsprings are put in
action early in the long game of life, in which we win our highest
natural privilege — our consciousness. And no wonder that this
vision-making process requires constant updating with reality inputs and frequent rebalancing in the repair shop of our dreams.

CHAPTER 9

The Heart of the Brain-Mind:
Emotion and Instinct

A YOUNG WOMAN named Sally, who lived in Boston, told me about a dream she had recently had.

I am on a bus in a large metropolis, and although it is daytime, I am uneasy and afraid of my surroundings. The people on the bus are all strangers, and I know that they do not notice me and would not like me or help me if I needed them. I am sitting in the front of the bus, on the right side, facing the aisle. A person in a wheelchair is in front of me, and I feel that he is crowding me. Although the bus is full, I notice a man in the back who frightens me. He looks like Charles Manson [the psychopath who used drugs and sex to enslave, torture, and maim young women]. Although the man does not look at me, I know that he is aware of me.

When the bus stops to let off the guy in the wheelchair, I look away, and when I look back, the man has moved forward one or two seats. He is reading a newspaper, and he doesn't move. When I look again, he is even closer, although I am not aware of him moving. I begin to panic. When he is two seats away, I try to get off the bus, but the driver will not open the door. I begin to cry in fear to an older woman in another seat, but she is annoyed and doesn't answer me. I am afraid to look at him, for fear he will look back. I scream and start to beat on the door of the bus, but nobody seems to believe me, and with my back turned I wait for the inevitable cold touch of his hand on my shoulder.

Sally's dream suggests that life in a modern metropolis might not be all that much safer than in the primitive jungle of our reputedly savage forebears. Then I told Sally a story of my own.

I was walking in a residential, downtown section of Boston in the wee hours of the morning, when three drug-crazed men suddenly appeared at my side. Once my assailants had cornered me, my sense of threat was of nightmarish intensity. Fear dominated my thinking. The most agonizing aspect of my dread was the sense that I was helpless and alone, even though I was surrounded by people. I knew that eyewitnesses to an urban assault would do nothing to help. One of the men tapped my shoulder to distract my attention, setting up a crippling cross-chop that knocked me down to the pavement and temporarily out. When I regained consciousness and looked up at my three assailants stomping me with their feet, I screamed as loudly in the Boston dawn as I could, but it was to no avail. No one bothered to get out of bed on that early spring morning, much less open a window, to verbally drive off my attackers or ask if I needed help.

Sally reacted knowingly to my account, until I told her that it wasn't a dream. I was the real-life victim of a brutal urban assault. I was beaten and bloodied and had screamed out to save my very life.

It is not surprising that young women who live in big cities have dream anxiety that matches the real thing. Sally didn't have my experience, she just anticipated it. But notice how well she anticipated it. Her emotions of fear, dread, anxiety, and panic, and her screaming out in complete terror, matched mine exactly. We could not have been in two more different states — she was in REM sleep, under domination of her cholinergic system and perceiving nothing from the outside world, and I was as awake and hyper-

aware of reality as my aminergic system could possibly make me —
yet our emotions were identical.

It is clear from this comparison that emotion is not just a way
of reacting to life's events. It is also created from within, and with
just as much intensity when it is spontaneous (as in Sally's dream)
as when it arises in response to a real threat. Emotion is a constant,
a fundamental part of all our brain-mind states. For Sally, it is as
if she came into the world equipped with the capacity to anticipate
the worst and rehearse for it in the throes of her Charles Manson
dream.

Anxiety is natural and healthy. And there is nothing necessarily
neurotic about it. Anxiety, however unpleasant, often serves us
well. My intuitive reflection on this recognition is that the brain is
an anxiety emitter. Like the heart, it beats constantly. As our emotional heart beats, it emits just enough unease to keep us wary.
After all, it is often wise to be wary. The brain-mind also emits just
enough of the other colors of the emotional rainbow to keep us
joyful enough, angry enough, sad enough, guilty enough, and
ashamed enough to live our lives with safety, gusto, and responsibility.

What are emotions? Where do they come from? What are they
good for? And how can it be that Sally and I, in such different
states, can have the exact same emotional experience?

WHY SCIENCE HAS SHUNNED EMOTION

When we say that our emotions are "primitive," we recognize
their long and important history in our rise from the evolutionary
swamp. But by calling emotions "primitive" we also tend to devalue their utility. As rationalists most of us are almost embar-
rassed by emotion. Like *Star Trek*'s Mr. Spock, we suppose that if
we were really sensible we wouldn't have to have any feelings at all.
It is no surprise, then, to find that science, being rational, has had
a very difficult time dealing with the subject of emotion. Why is it
so important for science to face the facts of our passions? Because
they not only influence our thoughts, they also constitute an im-

portant way of knowing the world that is independent of our intellect.

The psychoanalysts must be given enduring credit for always giving emotion their highest priority. But that admirable group of caretakers has had little more success in formulating a scientifically valid theory of emotions than the hardheaded experimentalists. As in so many other areas, the influence of Freud has held the field back intellectually. Freud's mistaken notion of how dreams are actually constructed contaminates the rest of his theory of mental life. For Freud, dreaming was a fundamentally neurotic process and a threat to our mental health. Censorship was needed to protect our pristine consciousness from the villainous, instinctual forces of the unconscious. And our dream emotions — especially anxiety — were a sure sign of the inadequacy of our defenses against our instinctual selves.

We need now to find a new way of looking at emotion, this ancestral, important, and essential part of ourselves. We need to recognize that emotion is itself an instinct and, as such, is crucial to our survival.

As long as all forms of spontaneous activity of the brain-mind went unrecognized by science, emotion could hardly have been expected to be seen for what it is: a constant flow of vital data from deep within ourselves. Once we adopt the idea that the brain-mind is a unified, dynamic system that manifests itself in a continuously varied sequence of activation states, we have no problem with the concept of emotion as one of its most reliable and useful products. The noun *emotion* stems from the verb *emote*, which means "to move away from; to move." Just as perception, which is driven by motor programs, is spontaneous as well as reactive, so too is emotion.

Another major obstacle to progress in understanding emotion has been the scientific taboo on subjective experience. Although many scientists had no difficulty with documenting behavioral aspects of emotional expression — like smiling or frowning — and finding out what stimuli produced these responses, the idea of using the attendant feelings themselves as data was anathema. The familiar objections included "can't be verified" and "too liable to distortion by suggestion or concealment." These complications may make experimentation difficult, but they certainly can be reduced to tolerable levels by smart collection and analysis of data.

The other main obstacle to seeing emotion as an essential building block of our conscious states was simply ignorance. Until we were well into the twentieth century we simply didn't know enough about the brain to speculate about how it might generate the emotional aspects of all our states. Now that we do, we can develop a testable theory of emotion. We must expect some surprises when the data starts to roll in, but if we don't have a theory that recognizes the ubiquity and spontaneity of emotion, we won't know what to look for. I will argue that subjective data is not only admissible but positively indispensable in exploring brain-mind states.

One way to get to the source and nature of emotions is through a careful study of REM sleep. Dreaming shows us that emotion is not just a way of reacting to life's events, but also an integral and useful part of our brain-mind states. And dreaming is perhaps more useful in its lucid revelation of emotion as a central building block of consciousness than it is for any other faculty. Precisely because it occurs when we are not reacting to the outside world, dream emotion provides the scientist with a powerful investigative tool for better understanding its mechanisms and functions.

WHAT IS EMOTION?

We're all familiar with the painful experience of fear that we have in our nightmares. But just flip a switch somewhere in our brain-mind and a dream becomes a completely different emotional scenario:

> I am walking down to a beachfront where in a short period of time I am flying (on my own accord) high in the sky, dipping down to "Nantucket," which is clear in my vision from above. This place I call Nantucket is a small island. I am feeling elated and free as I take high dives, circling up and down. A woman is reminding me to hurry so that I can catch the ferry back (back to where?). I minimize her concern as I notice how aqua and shimmery the water is

as I fly. This feeling is one that I do not want to end. I finally get
back to land; however, I don't recall landing. I read the ferry schedule, which indicates a 7:31 P.M. departure. My watch shows 7:25
P.M. I have a way to walk and don't think I can make it on time. I
am walking through local stores on my way, only because they are
in my path. I go through a Mexican store which has home furnish-
ings on sale up to 50 percent off. I take note of the many rugs hung
over one another. I finally reach the ferry landing but see the ferry
taking off in the distance. I am not concerned, even though it is the
last ferry of the evening.

This flying dream that was so enjoyed by my ecstatic informant,
Carol, could rightly be called a sensational high. Just as Sally wants
desperately to get off her dream bus, Carol wants to stay on her
dream flight. She is as invulnerable as a hawk as she soars above
Nantucket. And in the same way that our unpleasantly anxious
dreams prepare us for threatening situations, our ecstatic dreams
equip us for the elation and joy of life. The visual, motor, and emotional domains are as tightly linked in Carol's dream as they are
in Sally's.

Sally's and Carol's dreams are two from a large sample collected
in an experiment I designed with my colleague Jane Merritt to
identify and measure dream emotion. We found that negative and
positive emotions can be equally strong in dreams, but that negative emotions are far more frequent. Once each subject had written
out a dream report, we asked him or her to identify the emotions
present in each line of the report and to estimate the strength of
the emotions on a scale of one to three. Sally rated the emotion
"fear-anxiety" as 3+ for the lines during which Charles Manson
is moving toward her and for the line during which she is beating
on the door of the bus and screaming. Likewise, the score Carol
gave herself for "joy-elation" was 3+ for the line during which she
was dipping and diving and for the line during which she was having her psychedelic vision of the water.

In designing the study, we had to address several hotly debated
questions, which I will try to answer here. The first is: What is
emotion?

Everyone knows that emotion is what we feel. It is first and foremost a self-signal: a communication from one part of our brain-mind to another. Emotion helps us answer the banal question "How are you?" with more honesty to ourselves than is usually socially acceptable in our discourse with others. Most of us answer "Fine" when a friend asks "How are you?" even if we would really rather say "Downright depressed" (if we are sad or guilty) or "On top of the world" (if we are happy or elated).

Two other powerful emotions that we usually do not acknowledge openly are anxiety and anger. It is not often that a friend will reply to your "How are you?" with "Intolerably anxious, thank you." Anxiety is such a constant aspect of waking consciousness that we usually say "Fine" if our anxiety level is anything less than overwhelming panic. We don't like to communicate anger, either, because we don't want to offend a solicitous friend and because we are loath to admit that we harbor such potentially hurtful feelings. We also often prefer to conceal even strongly positive feelings like affection and sexual attraction. Most people aren't prepared for a response like "Extremely cuddly" or "Horny as a goat" when they ask casually, "How are you?"

Sometimes, however, we cannot conceal our feelings, no matter how hard we try. Even when we fail to get the messages ourselves, other people can often pick them up. "What's bugging you today?" a friend will ask you. "Oh, nothing," you reply, thinking to yourself, "It is *that* obvious?"

Thus we see that emotion is not only a signal to ourselves. It is a behaviorally coded message to others about our brain-mind states. Emotions communicate our availability, our approachability, and our affability in a language that is often more clear and direct than our words. In intimate relationships there is no place to hide from emotion. Emotion is the stuff that intimate relationships are made of.

Seen this way, emotion is a very important aspect of our brain-mind state. It determines our socially and biologically critical conjunctions and disjunctions. Our spectrum of emotions — the strength of the signals we emit in the various keys of our feelings — is nothing less than what we call personality. If we want to understand anything important about ourselves, we simply must take our emotions seriously.

How many different emotions are there? Most scholars usually come up with a list of six to twelve. When we asked the people in our dream emotion study to identify emotions, we had them choose from a list of seven: anger, anxiety-fear, shame-guilt, sadness, joy-elation, affection-eros, and surprise.

Any emotion inventory is liable to be incomplete. For example, we left "disgust" off our list because there is disagreement over whether it is indeed an emotion. Disgust is easily identifiable by someone's facial expression, one of the key signals of our emotional state. But others argue that disgust is a reflex response that requires a specific stimulus — like a bad smell. And at the higher level of, for example, displeasure with bad factions of society, disgust appears to require more conscience than most of us can easily muster in our dreams.

We did include "surprise," which is also a debated category. To me surprise has more to do with the orienting response than with emotion; I see it as a recognition of the novelty of, or inconsistency in, the flow of data we're receiving, rather than an evaluation of the data. Once we evaluate a surprise, our emotional reaction to it falls into one of the other categories, say, of fear or joy.

WHERE DO EMOTIONS COME FROM?

Facial expressions, body language, and more dramatic actions such as the pounding heart and sweaty palms of anxiety clearly indicate that emotional states are conveyed to — and through — the body. But are these bodily changes necessary for us to feel our emotions? If so, does emotion actually reside in our bodies? Or does it have a central aspect that is independent of our bodies?

William James, the American philosopher who tried in the 1890s to formulate an integrated theory of the brain and mind, thought that many of the bodily events that were mediated by our autonomic nervous system were read by our brain-mind as emotion. The autonomic nervous system controls our heart, blood vessels, stomach, and other organs (but not our muscles). While it is certainly true that stomach contractions and rapid heartbeat often signal anxiety, it now seems clear that these bodily sensations are neither necessary nor sufficient for us to feel anxious. Think for a moment about your most terrifying dreams and ask yourself if, in the grip of a nightmare, you are aware of your heart, stomach, or any other visceral organ. I am not.

Of course, a polygraphic recording of Sally's Charles Manson dream might have shown an increased heart rate, a rise in blood pressure, and respiratory irregularity. But Sally didn't feel these peripheral expressions of her emotion because all bodily sensations are actively blocked during REM sleep. She might also have had exactly the same bodily changes during quite a different dream.

When we dream, the brain stem sends two parallel messages to the spinal cord: one says no output (you can't move), and the other says no input (you can't feel). Further evidence that dream emotion does not depend on the body comes from dream reports. In these reports there is always a dramatic and total absence of descriptions of the bodily sensations of emotion. In her description of her terror during the Manson dream, Sally does not say that she was suddenly aware of breathing rapidly, feeling palpitations, or sweating as Manson edged nearer and nearer. Why not? Because she didn't sense those signals. She felt terror, as an emotion, inside her own brain-mind, and was completely unaware of her body.

Physiology finally did in James's theory of emotion. Charles Sherrington, the champion of the reflex doctrine, and Walter Cannon both showed that animals were fully capable of emotional behavior after the nerves to and from the body were cut. Emotions could be triggered simply by stimulating the brain.

Once Cannon had satisfied himself and the scientific world that signals from the body were not necessary for spontaneous emotion, he and Philip Bard set out to localize the central site of emotion in the brain. They showed they could induce emotions like fear and rage in animals by stimulating either the hypothalamus or the amygdala. And when the amygdala was removed, the animals were rendered tame, placid, and even docile.

We have since come to the same conclusion using more modern research — that the amygdala is an important brain center of emotion. Not only that, the neurons of the amygdala beat constantly: thus we produce emotions in all states, no matter how normal or bizarre.

Genetics probably sets an individual range of emotions within us, just as it sets the range of our pulses and blood pressures. We are the particular people that we are in large part because of the way our brain's emotion registers are set. We can tune this register to a degree as we mature from childhood, but the emotional music that is played out of us as personality is as distinctive as our fingerprints. When the volume is low, we are the only ones who hear this music. But turn the volume up and the whole world knows what state we are in. The amygdala is also like a player piano in that it runs through its own scores every day. Dreaming is an emotional recital: all stops are out and the keys are hammering away.

It is sad that so little scientific work on emotion is being done today. This lament is well sung by Joseph Le Doux at Cornell Medical School, one of the few brave scientists who has stayed with this critical scientific problem. Le Doux points out that the recent growth of cognitive science, while restoring consciousness to its rightful place within psychology, has tended to explain away emotion as a merely cognitive process.

While it is certainly true that emotion and cognition are integrated, they are not one and the same. Sally feels Charles Manson coming close to her before she sees him. In her dream, it seems possible that the cognitive perceptions — the images of Manson she sees when she *does* look back — may have been generated by her brain to account for her mounting sense of dread. Once again, the brain is concocting a story to link the random firing of the brain's neurons, in this case not to make sense of images, *but to create images to make sense of emotions.* Evidence that emotion and cognition are not one was also apparent during my awakening at the Columbus hotel, when my misperception of the clinking sound outside my bedroom caused anxiety, which in turn caused me to have even more radical misperceptions.

The study of dream emotion has already allowed us to conclude that the brain is an emitter of feelings. Whether we are scientific rationalists trying to tune out emotion in order to free our cognition from the bias of sentiment, or romantic artists trying to tune up our emotions to drown out the nagging voice of rationality, the fundamental reality of emotion is the same. Emotion is not just a reaction to the world, it is a spontaneous and constantly present component of our subjective experience, and of ourselves, that others pick up, read, and describe as our personalities. The body conveys emotion as it amplifies and channels the signals of our emotional states, but emotion is an integral and independent aspect of all activated brain-mind states. By looking more closely at dream emotion we can expect to greatly advance our understanding of this basic aspect of human nature.

FEAR MORE THAN JOY

What is the nature of our spontaneous emotion spectrum as it is revealed in dreaming? It will come as no surprise to most dreamers that anxiety is the leading batter in the lineup of dream emotions. The subjects of our dream emotion experiment produced 200 dream reports, and after we had asked them to identify the types of emotions they felt, if any, line for line in the reports, we computed the average incidence of the various emotions indicated. Anxiety had the highest batting average of .321; of the 809 incidences of emotion indicated in the reports, 260 of them were notations of anxiety or fear. Joy-elation was solidly in second place with an average of .255. This means that well over half of all dream emotions (57 percent) are extreme; our emotional state tends to tilt one way or the other so that dreams are either pleasant or unpleasant.

This tilt is much more frequently toward the unpleasant, however, because anger is strongly in third place on the list. When adding up all the incidences of emotion, the total proportion of unpleasant emotions comes to 68.1 percent — a little more than two-thirds. When a friend wishes us "pleasant dreams," we should be aware that we have, on average, only a one in three chance of having one. Surely this finding negates Freud's idea that dreams are a fulfillment of wishes.

The weakest hitter on the dream team is affection-eros, whose average was a lowly .064. A batter with this kind of performance risks being traded to the Pony League! And taken together, the positive emotions — joy, elation, affection, and eros — comprise only 31.9 percent of the entire spectrum.

We were not the first dream scientists to come up with this important information. Three previous studies had shown the same general profile. What *was* newly revealing about our study, however, was the quantity of emotions. By asking subjects to score their own reports, we obtained an incidence of emotion that was ten times higher than that reported in previous studies. That is because when people are simply asked to give dream reports, they spend an inordinate amount of time describing the plot and the visions, not the emotions. But when you ask them to go back and ponder what they were feeling as they experienced those events, then they note their emotions in much more detail. Clearly, our brain-mind is emitting some emotion almost all the time in this state.

The increase in the sensitivity of our dream-emotion measuring technique, while encouraging, gives us pause because we don't really have any direct way of knowing how much emotion is with us in the dream state, or in the waking state for that matter. How much of what kind of emotion are you feeling right now? We simply do not yet have enough valid data about how our emotions are actually perceived in any of our conscious states. More careful examination of the issue is needed.

We also need more precise and objective measures. At present, we have no idea how the amygdala or its related temporal lobe structures mediate the different emotions. Le Doux's animal work suggests that fear is mediated by the nucleus of the amygdala, but neither he nor anyone else has looked at any of the other emotions with the powerful anatomical and physiological techniques that are now available. And emotion may be one fundamental faculty that is too tough to solve using only animal models.

Now that we have the new imaging methods for mapping brain activation in humans we can begin this work. The imaging machines or scanners are familiar to most of us who have had computerized X-ray pictures taken for diagnostic purposes. Suppose that Sally had her Charles Manson nightmare, or that Carol had her

Nantucket flying dream, while sleeping with her head in a brain imaging machine. It's almost as easy to fall asleep in some types of brain scanner as it is to nod off in one of those metal beehives at the hairdresser's. Suppose, for that matter, that we could capture and compare Bertal's fear and flight from the dive-bombers with my fear and flight from my woodshed helper. My question is this: Would the emotional brain activity associated with the dreams of Sally and Carol (which had opposite but extreme emotions), or the states of Bertal and me (which had the same emotions but in different states), be similar or different? And could scanners sense a difference if there was one? We will soon know. Indeed, a colleague of mine at Harvard has himself slept in a brain scanner, and the emotion center in his brain, his amygdala, lit up the night during REM sleep. Now we must find ways to use this and other powerful new tools analytically.

AH MEN! AH WOMEN!

I occasionally appear as a guest on talk shows, and callers frequently ask: "Are the dreams of men different from those of women?" They would like me to come up with something that will fit their widely held stereotypes about gender difference: We all know that women are more emotional than men, don't we? And being maternal, they express affection more freely, don't they? They are a less angry lot than hypercompetitive males, right?

Wrong! When it comes to dream emotion, the answers to all these questions is no. We found *no* significant difference between men and women on any measure of dream emotion. The actual figures for men versus women were so similar they are not worth listing.

How do we explain this? The answer may be that, deep down, we're *not* all that different emotionally. I believe that Darwin's conclusion that our emotional repertoire is the result of our adaptive capability should be taken very seriously. The full spectrum of emotion is likely to be shared by all members of a species regardless of their sex.

It is also clear that men and women have exactly the same range of brain-mind states, with the exception of minor fluctuations in association with the menstrual cycle and major disruptions of sleep during pregnancy. No gender differences have been reported in the study of any major sleep-wake variable. This implies that the REM-sleep activation mechanism, down to its cells and chemical messages, is identical in both sexes. Turn it on and out come the same emotions for men and women, in the same relative proportions.

Will we have the same surprise when more scientists begin to look at emotions in the waking state? It seems likely to me. That doesn't mean that biology has nothing to do with sex-role differentiation. Men are bigger and stronger (on average) and women bear the children (well above the average), so we need to be cautious about pushing the concept of gender sameness too far. Nonetheless, it does appear that the REM-sleep state reveals an internal sounding board whose emotional notes, when struck by the amygdala in the player-piano mode, makes strikingly similar music in both sexes.

One strong part of the dream-emotion message is that feelings are important components of the activated brain-mind states of all people. A second is that the spectrum of emotion is strongly shifted to the negative side and this skew is shared by men and women. The power of positive thinking thus has a lot to compete with! Why are we set up this way? What are the benefits of experiencing life with such worry and violent feelings?

WHAT ARE EMOTIONS GOOD FOR?

If Charles Darwin were not so well known as the author of *Origin of Species,* his book entitled *The Expression of Emotions in Man and Animals* would probably be much more widely recognized and appreciated. Darwin clearly recognized that emotions are important signals that accurately communicate the brain-mind state of one animal to another. When confronted with a stranger, the first response is an internal alerting that says, "Orient: stop, look and listen!" This is followed with strong body signals made so that any intruder can read them: hairs rise, ears go up, eyes widen, and movement is frozen. The intruder is put on notice that he has been identified and is being critically evaluated: Are you friend or foe?

These bodily changes are not only preparation for further evaluation of threat (the sensory aspect of emotion), but they simultaneously prepare us for an active motor response. The most conservative response is flight — escape — which is served by increasing blood flow to the muscles. Heart action increases, blood pressure rises, and respiratory rate goes up. If escape is impossible and a showdown becomes inevitable, the same physiology serves the preparation for a fight.

This initial reaction is what Walter Cannon later called the fight-or-flight response, and he showed that its physiology was mediated by the sympathetic nervous system, the subset of the autonomic nervous system that controls the heart, blood vessels, and lungs. We now know that this sympathetic activation includes strong signals carried by the aminergic system of the brain stem, which prepare the brain-mind for action by heightening all the functions normally associated with waking. Norepinephrine and serotonin are the bells of the brain's own internal alarm system.

As we become alert we can process data faster and evaluate it more critically because our brain-minds are more highly activated. At the same time, we become more precisely oriented. Not only are we better at analysis, we are far more likely to remember threatening encounters and all their associated parameters for future reference. This is because we are not only sensitized for the short term, but instructed for the long term.

Our capacity to do this is built in. That is precisely what we mean by the word *instinctual*. According to the brain-mind paradigm, anxiety, coupled with arousal, is an *instinctual emotional capacity* that operates at some finite level all the time. Anxiety is the leading emotion because it is the most important emotion; there is no way that anxiety can be regarded as secondary or as derived from sexual and aggressive instincts, as Freud assumed. Anxiety is healthy, and it is an indispensable tool of our survival.

Whether to flee or to fight is a decision that follows, perhaps automatically. And it is one that our dreams help us rehearse.

When Charles Manson edged nearer and nearer to Sally, she froze and prepared to flee, because she was trapped and knew she couldn't win the fight. I reacted in the same way when I was cornered by the junkies, for the same reasons.

Sally's nightmare ended as she pounded, screaming, on the bus door. She might have pummeled Manson if her dream state had not been interrupted by the massive arousal that activated her cortex and woke her up. I wonder how many times my own brain-mind had been preparing me with nightmares for my real showdown in the street. I never took boxing lessons, I never took judo, but I knew, procedurally, how to fight when it became clear that my life depended on it.

Fortunately, such showdowns can usually be avoided. But when they become inevitable, it is important to know what to do to try to mitigate them. As Darwin recognized, two things serve to reduce the occurrence of damaging interaction. One is the signaling of fear and appeasement or submission by either party; the reciprocal is the signaling of readiness to fight, perhaps accompanied by an advisory indicating the terms of a peaceful settlement.

We would all rather be cozy, warm, and sexually gratified than scared stiff or fighting mad. And we know how to do these things too. We just have to be careful about whom we do them with, and where and when — which narrows the list of prospects considerably. It seems our brain-mind states are designed conservatively in this crucial emotional area. We approach one another with a circumspection and caution that is born of our existential fear and anxiety, and bred in the bristles of our anger and aggression. Narrow is the gate. Maybe it's because it is so very sweet, so hard to get, and so very hard to hold on to that we keep affection and eros in such high esteem.

REHEARSING OUR LIVES

The Darwinian revolution in biology has branched into two main pathways. One, the better traveled, is called molecular genetics. This pathway is just converging with brain-mind theory, in the idea that REM sleep provides a time, a place, and the appropriate chemistry to combine our genetic instructions with our experiential data. The other, called ethology, looks at behavior in terms of the goals of survival and procreation.

Ethology assumes that many behaviors, such as mating rituals, nest building, and territorial defense, have a genetically built-in action program. When activated by the appropriate stimulus, such as an attractive female, a baby's cry, or a competitive male, the action program then sets the appropriate behaviors in motion. Innate behaviors have several defining properties: they occur without training; they are more likely to occur if the interval between the last occurrence has been long; and they have an all-or-none quality — once they have commenced they tend to run to completion.

Feeding and drinking are easily understood examples. They both have high survival value. They don't have to be learned. They seem never to be forgotten, even in the depth of dementia. The longer it has been since the last consumption, the more likely they are to occur. Feeding and drinking are also state-dependent. They frequently occur together in waking but are markedly underrepresented in dreaming.

Feeding-and-drinking and sleep-and-dreaming could thus be viewed as two mutually exclusive survival strategies. Instead of investing energy in seeking water and food, the organism sleeps to conserve both water and calories by reducing activity and exposure. And consider this: hunger and thirst are both regulated by the hypothalamus, the very same part of the brain that tells us when to sleep and when to wake. Perhaps this is why the French say "Qui dort, dine," meaning, "When we sleep, we eat!"

Ethologists now theorize that the brain stem is the seat of the programs for many of these fixed acts. We have already encountered this idea in our consideration of motor-pattern generators. We conclude that sleep is itself an instinct. And it contains within it the operation of the central program for three other instincts, namely: the anxiety and orienting responses that serve survival by alerting us to danger; the anger and aggression that ready us to repel attackers and to fight for our lives if necessary; and the sexual arousal that promotes affection, affiliations, and the consummation of desire that is essential to our future as a species.

Ethologists will have no difficulty in appreciating the functional importance of our daily round of brain-mind states. REM sleep is appetitive: if we are prevented from sleeping, we experience an increased drive to sleep; any losses incurred are promptly and precisely repaid. REM sleep is fixed: the automatic activation of the brain-mind in REM sleep guarantees the running of instinct programs so that they will always be practiced and thus available when needed. Furthermore, REM sleep allows these programs to be updated with new experiential data. This is why dreaming so clearly reflects the where, when, and with whom aspects of our instinctively driven emotional interactions.

Emotion complements our memory by giving it a valence: how we really feel about this person or that, this experience or that, this place or that. Emotion is a way not only of perceiving, but also of orienting to the world. It is a way of being strongly tied to purposes so dark and deep that were it not for their glorious unveiling in our dreams we might go through life pretending they were not there. In dreaming there is no place to hide from our instinctual selves and from our biological destinies.

CHAPTER 10

Stop, Look, and Listen: Attention and Distraction

MY FRIEND Kaji Asó is a man of many talents. Besides being a master of classical Japanese brush painting, he sings Italian opera with glass-shattering force and heart-warming brio. As if this weren't enough, he is also able to entertain the child in each of us with his parlor magic. Each trick in Kaji's repertoire depends on sleight of hand: he pulls from his right ear the Ping-Pong ball that he has just put in his mouth, and makes a white napkin mouse jump from his palm to his elbow. Kaji is able to perform these magic acts by purposefully misdirecting the viewer's attention and implanting erroneous expectations in the viewer's brain-mind.

No matter how many times Kaji repeats his tricks, they fool us. To say that "the hand is quicker than the eye" misses the point, however. Kaji's hands don't move that fast. And they are always — or almost always — in full view. Kaji's manual speed is not the essence of his deception. It is the provision of false cues about what to expect next that catches our attention and commits us to an expectation that the magician can sneak behind. When P. T. Barnum said, "There's a sucker born every minute," he was noting that our attentional system is ready to be fooled by misleading cues at every minute of our lives.

One of the surest ways of knowing that you have free will is to notice your ability to select what you pay attention to, to select the information that occupies your mind. This ability to selectively attend, however, is complicated by the noise and turmoil of the world around us and by the surge of emotions and thoughts that arise continuously from within us. Our ability to attend or to be distracted depends as much on these internal forces as it does on outside stimuli. The decision to focus, to concentrate, and to select and direct our thoughts requires an almost herculean effort. I maintain that it is the very essence of willpower to think along certain lines and to abandon others. All that is most gloriously human is dependent upon our capacity to direct our consciousness. It is essential to art, science, learning, and the moral fabric of our lives.

This will is not always easy to enact, however. I relearn this every autumn at my farm in Vermont. When the weather suddenly changes from sultry to brisk, the local flies make an aggressive effort to enter the warm house and feed on any part of my anatomy that is exposed. Just the other day, while I was putting the finishing touches on an oil painting, the pernicious little monsters began to attack my ankles. They destroyed my eye-hand coordination by sending distracting signals to my brain. Which should I attend to, the paintbrush or the flies? No way I could deal with both, and no way I could deny the existence of the distraction. Perhaps a practiced Buddhist meditator could have maintained focus, but not I. My Western brain is best when it is attending to one channel of data at a time. I had to put down the brush and whisk them away. I couldn't stand it.

So how do we negotiate the tug of war between attention and distraction? How do we select the signals we want to focus on and exclude the distracters? Why do we sometimes become obsessed with a thought or deed, and how do we later break free from it? Why are we so focused in the morning, but continually more easily distracted as the day wears on? And how is it that we can process information from our environment in the foreground of our minds, while also processing the memories, plans, and references that comprise the necessary context in the background? Let us use some of the brain chemistry and the AIM model presented in Part One to explain our ability to attend or to be distracted and how this ability varies in different states.

FOCUSING OUTWARD OR INWARD

We all know how fragile our ability to pay attention can be. When we have lost even a little sleep, attention is the faculty that flags first: we have trouble staying with our tasks; we are distracted by insignificant stimuli; and our minds wander from topic to topic and from fantasy to reality. We lose our ability to stay on track, to maintain our direction toward a goal, and even to feel calm.

In order to pay attention, we must keep a constant fix on the bandwidth of data we are processing and on its external or internal source. Paying attention not only requires strong will, but commits our brain-mind's resources to a restricted set of targets. Paying attention to one thing means necessarily ignoring many others. It drains mental energy and entails an experiential sacrifice.

The flip side is that attention can become involuntarily locked onto its target. We become obsessed rather than distracted, and our behavior is compulsive rather than aimless. Upon leaving our house for a trip, the idea that we have left our tickets behind is so strong that we have to check again and again that we have them. If we are lucky, some part of us notices that we are overly concerned and frees us from a fruitless reaffirmation of the obvious.

Attention, then, must remain centered in dynamic tension between distraction and obsession if our behavior is to stay on a moderate course.

The sensory data that compete for our attention are myriad, and our selection task is, at every instant, formidable. We have eight modalities to choose from: the five senses — vision, hearing, touch, taste, smell — and three data channels that come from within our bodies — posture, movement, and pain. That's the bad news. The good news is that we can do it. First we prioritize the millions of bits of data that knock on the doors of our consciousness from dawn until dusk, and then we decide what to make of the bits that are admitted.

To better enjoy a kiss we close our eyes. In doing so, we exclude the normally huge demand that vision puts on our processing capability and devote more of our resources to the subtle, tactile experience of kissing. Once the act is under way, sensual pleasure may, for some, be enhanced by reopening the eyes and admitting visions that enhance arousal. The first process is one of fine-tuning the input, like zeroing in on a radio station on your stereo. The second is one of enhancing intensity, like adding a second pair of speakers to increase the volume and depth of the music.

Increasing pleasure and decreasing pain are among the immediate benefits of sensory channel selection. I used to dread going to the dentist until I discovered just how well I could train myself to select the contents of consciousness. Now I anticipate my time in that erstwhile torture chamber by loading up my neuronal networks with alternative inputs. When the drilling starts, I never close my eyes or tense my muscles, both of which are sure to make the pain and anxiety worse. Instead I gaze up at the sky through the window and imagine the sunlit scene on Crane's Beach in Ipswich or visualize the fall-painted woods behind my place in Vermont.

Notice that in this act of dental dissociation, I have done more than just select the data channel. I have switched input sources from external to internal. And I have shifted away from the foreground of external sensory data processing and toward the background of internal mental activity that we call fantasy. I am well on my way to the brain-mind state commonly known as hypnosis, a subject to which we will return in Part Three.

There is still another kind of attentional freedom to consider. I can change the mode and strength of the internal representations that occupy my consciousness. The quality and intensity of the mental activity that we call fantasy can vary from exclusively verbal, through partially visual, to intensely hallucinatory. The degree to which my consciousness attends to data from the outside world or from my own thoughts is widely variable.

By changing focus from external to internal, we are moving toward the domain of dreaming and psychosis. Attention, like all other faculties of the brain-mind, is state dependent. One key variable is volition. I can voluntarily shift attention only when I am awake. In sleep my attention is riveted to internally generated data. Since we now know that the state shift from waking to sleeping is achieved by the brain stem, we might better understand attention itself by exploring those bottom-up processes that shift it. Because attention has a strongly voluntary aspect, we might also learn how to gain some top-down control over the bottom-up processes that govern our brain-mind states. The payoff would then come from finding natural and scientifically valid ways to manage our consciousness via the selective action of attention. Self-hypnosis, pain control, and the plain old power of positive thinking are among the prizes that we seek.

MEASURING ATTENTION

The behavioral signs of attention are easily measured, and the data constitutes a leading edge of the renaissance in cognitive science. One scientist who has been particularly successful in analyzing attention is Michael Posner of the University of Oregon.

In one of his schemes, Posner uses careful measurements of reaction time to reconstruct the sequence of brain-mind events that underlie our attentive behavior. A person is asked to fix his gaze on a spot of light in the center of a computer screen. (Electrodes placed just above the eyelids determine compliance with this restriction.) While the subject's gaze is fixed, Posner will flash a dot of light to the right or left side of the screen. The subject is to indicate his recognition of the dot's appearance as quickly as possible by pressing the appropriate key on the computer keyboard. The computer then calculates the time elapsed between the activation of the target on the screen and the subject's manual response.

Imagine how you would feel if you were seated at Posner's computer. No matter how laid back you believe yourself to be, something in you wants to do this task well. You want to be quick. And you may even want to figure out a way to beat the system. You are quite alert (and even a bit anxious) as you await the dot.

To whet your appetite, Posner will sometimes provide you with a cue as to which side of the screen the next signal will appear. Other times the cue will not contain a directional hint. But to prevent you from jumping the gun, the intervals between trials are unpredictably varied. But that's not all. The test is even more diabolical in that only 80 percent of the directional cues Posner gives you will be accurate; 20 percent will be misleading. When the arrow points to the right, the target will actually appear on the left, or vice versa. Finally, the sequence of cues — valid, invalid, or missing — will be randomized.

As you can imagine, your reaction time will be faster when you are given a valid cue to the target's location than when you are given a neutral cue. And of course, it will take you longer still to recognize a target when it appears in the unexpected half of your visual space, because you will waste time searching in the wrong half of the screen before you switch over to the right half. Thus the reaction time for a correctly guided search is faster than that for a random search, which is faster than that for an incorrectly guided search. As other life endeavors have taught us, a wrong hypothesis is more costly than an open mind.

The difference in response time under the three cue conditions is considerable. If you are given a correct cue, your reaction time will on average be 85 milliseconds faster than if you are given no cue. This difference is referred to as the "benefit" of correctly anticipated attention. If you are misled by an invalid cue, your reaction time will be 36 milliseconds slower than if given no cue. That is the "cost" of incorrectly anticipated attention. The range is therefore $85 + 36 = 121$ milliseconds, or 1.21 tenths of a second, which could mean the difference between life and death if you were driving a car. Of course, the range would be much wider if you had enjoyed a two-martini lunch or if you were sleepy.

Although the basic reaction-time experiment is old hat in psychology, it gains enhanced power when used with new technology. Imaging techniques like the CAT scans now routinely used in hospitals, and PET and MRI scans now used in research, are dramatically revolutionizing cognitive science by showing us in real time what is happening in the brain. We are now able to visualize the activity of our brain-minds as we see a dog or search for random dots on a video screen. It is this technology that permits cognitive scientists like Posner to test their inferences about the sequences of brain activity that underlie attention.

By placing a subject's head in a positron-emission tomography (PET) scanner and injecting a radioisotope into the bloodstream, it is possible to obtain pictures of the brain-mind at work. Neurons that are active consume more blood sugar and oxygen than those that are inactive. The greater the activity, the greater the consumption. Thus the radioisotopes carried by the blood congregate in areas of high activity. The protons emitted by the isotopes from any region of the brain, sensed by the scanner, accurately reflect the net activity of the neurons in that region. The computer produces a brightly colored paint-by-number portrait of your brain-mind as you try to beat the system in the reaction-time game. The activated regions of the brain "light up" on the scanner's screen.

Using the PET scanner in conjunction with the reaction-time test and others, it has become clear that each aspect of attention involves a specific area of the cortex. When Posner flashes a dot on the screen, the posterior (rear) region of the cortex, where vision is processed, lights up first, followed by the central region of the cortex, where spatial analyses are formed. The anterior (forward) region of the cortex, where identification occurs, lights up third. Once the posterior system has answered the question "Where is it?" (left or right), the anterior system addresses the question "What is it?" (a dot).

These two questions have long been recognized as key stages in the processing of perceptual data. And we have already considered them in discussing the orienting response (where is it?) and orientation (what is it?). Orientation is mediated by the brain stem, and it should come as no surprise that cognitive scientists have determined that the brain stem also mediates attention.

In order for us to attend to either external or internal information, our brain-minds must be sufficiently activated And in order to hold any external or internal target in mind, we must be able to maintain that activation. As we noted in chapter 5, activation (A), input source (I), and modulation (M) all depend on the brain stem and the aminergic-cholinergic system.

Posner has developed an anatomical model of attention. In it, two upper-brain components (the posterior and the anterior cortex) are responsible for orienting to a signal and the orientation needed to localize that signal, and one lower-brain vigilance component (the brain stem) is responsible for activating and directing the two upper-brain components. Sound familiar? Indeed it does, but now the brain stem is running attention around our images of the outside world as they are being received, not later in a dream simulation of external reality. Of the three modulatory (M) chemicals, it is norepinephrine that is most essential for attention, according to Posner.

We can test this conclusion with self-observation. Norepinephrine levels fall whenever we become sleepy (or even bored); in these states we have difficulty focusing our attention. We lose sight of the words as we read a book at bedtime or lose sight of the road as we drive late at night. The cortex is not getting the juice it needs to stay "lit up." And recall that in dreams we are never able to stop the action to focus on some detail; our ability to attend is disabled. As we know, during dreaming, the cortex is missing norepinephrine and the control that it confers.

WATCHING OURSELVES DREAM . . . AND HALLUCINATE

With practice, in our dreams, we can call up just enough norepinephrine to give us some control. At rare times we experience what is called lucid dreaming — while still in a dream, we become aware we are dreaming. This awareness is usually fleeting and more often wakes us up. But we know, for an instant, we are dreaming. Certain individuals, like my colleague Ed Pace-Schott, can sometimes make themselves become lucid while dreaming. When he succeeds, he regains control of his attention. He does this in two ways. One is to notice and pay attention to the bizarre discontinuities and incongruities that label dreaming so clearly, instead of ignoring these obvious clues as we usually do. The second is to tell himself to make voluntary movements (that is, to seize control) of his eyes instead of letting them flit back and forth automatically as they usually do.

With some encouragement from Ed, I have renewed my interest in lucid dreaming. And I use a similar one-two punch. First I notice the obvious fact that I am dreaming, and then I will an act that corresponds to what I am seeing in my dreams. If I am flying, I tell myself to flap my arms.

My arms don't actually move in bed, but what I am doing is engaging in volition. I am purposely starting a motor program. My theory is that by doing this I am engaging my frontal cortex to call for chemical help. My brain stem responds by sending up some norepinephrine — just enough to place me on the knife's edge between REM sleep and waking. If I push the system too hard, I will wake up. If I let up a bit, I will become reabsorbed in the dream.

We could probably capture this on a brain scanner. Normally, the brain stem has the power over a dream, and the frontal cortex is trying to catch up by imposing a plot. But during lucid dreaming, the cortex has caught up and can begin to direct, or at least watch, the action from a distance, like directing or watching a movie. During lucid dreaming the frontal cortex should light up faintly, even if not enough to outshine the brain stem.

The fact that lucid dreaming is possible is not just amusing. It is extremely important, because it gives us a critical key to unlocking psychosis. We have already concluded that dreaming is a psychosis. It's just a healthy one. If the parallel holds, then people who are mentally ill should have lucid psychotic episodes too. And they do! Indeed, it is the first step toward recovery. When patients gain such insight, they finally realize they are psychotic. Although they will still suffer the effects of their illness, they can begin to take control.

Even Bertal, whose episodes were sometimes extreme, had moments of insight. Remember when I found him squatting on the floor, in the kitchen of The Psycho, cramped up in a ball? It was after his hallucinations, but before he regained control of his posture, that he said, "Why do I do the foolish things I do?" There were a few times when Bertal seemed to realize that his hallucinations and actions were unhealthy or harmful.

The power of lucid observation was demonstrated to me by Harriet North, a patient of mine at The Psycho in the 1960s. She too was psychotic, but had come to the realization that she had a problem and had found a way to begin to control it. When a hallucination began, she would try to picture her library at home. She would look at the imaginary shelves and start to count the books, focusing on each one as best she could as she counted. Soon, her hallucination would stop. Harriet's insight did not stop the psychosis, but the library trick did. The visualization and counting were voluntary motor acts; she directed her eyes at the books and carried out the rational exercise of counting. By doing both these things, she was imposing top-down control, which quashed the bottom-up hallucination signal. She was purposefully lighting up her cortex so that it drowned out her lower brain, snapping her out of her episode just as cognition wakes us up out of a dream.

CHANGING FOCUS AND PAYING ATTENTION

What happens when you look up from your book in response to a person who has just entered the room? You switch your attention.

That is not a simple matter for people who have had damage to the parietal lobe of their cortex, on the right side of their brains. These patients, who suffer from what is called hemi-neglect, have trouble disengaging and shifting their attention. They tend to become fixed on things in one half of visual space and to ignore the other half. For them the world has been cut in half, but they are completely unaware of their loss.

Engagement is controlled by the thalamus, a deep central structure in the brain. It projects messages widely to areas of the cortex and receives powerful feedback from each of them. Because of its central position and its reciprocal firing pattern, the thalamus is the ideal point at which to intercept unwanted or unexpected data. *Selective* attention depends as much on the suppression of irrelevant data as it does on the amplification of relevant data, and the thalamus is good at suppression. By feeding no-go signals into the thalamus, huge areas of the cortex can be effectively deprived of input. In an analogy to radio, the thalamus is a very effective tuning filter for the brain-mind.

We can see this directly in monkeys, who, happily, are able to learn to play Posner's reaction-time game. Monkeys perform these routine operations over and over for modest rewards such as a sip of juice. As they play the game, it is possible to record the activity in their brain cells to document the dramatic effects attention has on the neurons that process visual data. One of the most surprising revelations is that vision is "built up" within the brain as signals are processed via two distinct pathways from the posterior cortex forward toward the anterior cortex. How well these images are built up depends strongly on how closely the monkeys are paying attention.

Furthermore, when the monkeys (and we humans) shift attention, their cortex must disengage the current target and communicate with the thalamus to reengage on a new target. This sequence occurs flawlessly and thoughtlessly eight to ten times a second. Can you immediately disengage your attention from this book? Of course. Can you reengage on a person entering the room? Rapidly.

While we need to be able to engage and disengage our attention, we also need to be able to maintain our attention once we have focused on something. As a high school or college student your academic success was related to your ability to resist distraction, to pay sustained attention to your book no matter who walked into the room, such as the library, where you were studying. You had both a sharp focus and a sustained span of attention even when friends tempted you to talk or flirt instead of study. While you may have taken justifiable pride in your capacity to pay attention, you must admit that it would have been considerably more difficult had you lived in a society where every stranger might have been a member of the secret police. I suppose that's one reason it is so hard to make eye contact with native riders on the Moscow subway. For them, being watched has a sinister social implication.

Maintaining our attention, or deciding to switch it, depends on tuning in and out the many channels of input we receive and the many channels of output, such as motor commands, that we have at our disposal. Unnecessary noise in either direction uses up the limited resources of the attentional system.

"Tuning" seems to be just the right word to describe how the thalamus sustains the proper level of tension. Electronics engineers call this process signal sharpening. Several independent scientists now maintain that norepinephrine cells in the brain stem play a critical role in the tuning of attention. Norepinephrine increases the ratio of signal to noise.

This theory arose from neurophysiological studies of the listening capability of squirrel monkeys. Whenever the animals became inattentive or drowsy, there was a corresponding drop in activity of norepinephrine cells and presumably of the norepinephrine that was released in the brain stem, thalamus, and cortex. When we are "out of it," we aren't pushing our brain stem's norepinephrine supplier hard enough; when we are on the qui vive, we have this system working well for us; and when we are stressed out, we are pushing it too far.

LOSS OF VIGILANCE

We become drowsy, daydream, or become generally inattentive because our brains are producing less norepinephrine. This output is reduced to its lowest level during dreaming. And what happens to our capacity to attend in dreaming: Is our internal attention selective? Do we focus? Is our attentional span long? Can we think? Are we able to hold an idea or image in mind?

The answer to all these questions is no. Internal attention is lost during dreaming. I cannot control the images, feelings, ideas, or actions in my dreams. During my New Orleans hotel dream, when the security guard was trying to find intruders in the room above, I was far from focusing, fine-tuning, or evaluating. I was dissolved in a flood of sensations, emotions, and actions about which my ideas were decidedly flaky.

On the other hand, my associative capacities are never greater than in my dreams. I am awash in wildly uncritical and imaginative fabrications, which implies that the vast capabilities of my "what is it?" system are being brought to bear on whatever problem is suggested. While I don't believe that the evidence for real-life problem solving in dreams is very good, I am impressed by the motley array of tricks that my brain-mind trots out, as if to show them off or give them their daily exercise.

There are two good experimental ways to find out if my attentive difficulties during waking and dreaming are related to a lack of norepinephrine. One is to interfere with norepinephrine during waking by giving me a drug and seeing what happens to my performance on the Posner reaction-time task. The other is to wake me up from non-REM and REM sleep, put me immediately on Posner's machine, and compare my performance then to my performance during the day. Both tests have been done, and both produce the same results: the speed of disengagement from a target is faster when one is awakened from sleep than when one is awake during the day. Subjects disengage their attention unusually quickly when norepinephrine levels are low, which fits with our subjective experience of dreaming.

Rapid disengagement is not necessarily good, as shown by children who have attention deficit disorder. For decades the assumption about kids who didn't pay attention, particularly when in school, was that they were "hyperactive." This was the conclusion because the same kids were usually fidgeting, moving around in their chairs, and tapping their feet on the floor instead of staring in blurry-eyed obedience at the blackboard. Note that their "hyperactivity" consists of motor acts. Focusing their eyes on the blackboard and maintaining their concentration (volition) also depend on motor programs. The problem with such children is not that they can't pay attention to anything, it's that they are paying attention to everything. They rapidly disengage from a given signal in order to engage all the others. They fail to inhibit enough motor signals so they can focus on a few.

Today these children are put on a regimen of a mild amphetamine, a molecule that is similar to norepinephrine (notice that
amphetamine is an amine). This boost enables them to inhibit some
of the distracting motor movements, allowing them to concentrate
better. There are adults who have the same problem and are helped
with the same drugs.

The main point is that impairments in attention, whether they
occur in the REM-sleep state or the awake state of people with
attention deficit disorder, share a common chemical cause: a decrease in output from the norepinephrine system. At least we have
an experimental handle on the slippery issues of what sleep may do
to — and for — attention, and how those effects may be mediated.
This is a good case of how the brain-mind paradigm, in explaining
a faculty of a normal state, can be used to find a solution to a
problem with the same faculty in an abnormal state.

There is also an ethical point to be made here. The insight
gained with the brain-mind paradigm is important because it explains *why* a drug treatment works. Doctors have known for some
years now, based on clinical trials, that amphetamines help mediate
attention deficit disorder, but they haven't known why. This is dangerous. If we don't know the root cause of a problem, we can't
predict the effect of a treatment. It could well have been that the
amphetamines helped the children in the short term but aggravated
the problem in the long term. We simply couldn't predict if this was
so. Now we can be sure that it is not the case. Furthermore, it is
hard to find alternative treatments if we don't know the root cause
of a problem. Some children cannot tolerate the drugs. Once the
brain-mind theory explains why the disorder occurs, we can methodically and successfully find other treatments.

For example, it would have been very useful to have this understanding when I was trying to help Bertal. It is clear, now, that
Bertal shared some of the same symptoms as children who can't
select what to attend to and what to ignore. In giving his childhood
history to us at The Psycho, Bertal's mother described him as a
"misfit." His school record was poor, and in the ninth grade he was
dropped from school because of inattention in class and suspected
involvement in homosexual and fire-setting activities. Inattention

in class! What a clue! Unfortunately, this was in the 1950s, long before attention deficit disorder was recognized.

The brain-mind theory of inattention also could have helped us understand why chlorpromazine worked on Bertal. We gave him chlorpromazine to calm him down when he was reacting wildly to every input from his external and internal sources. We knew then that chlorpromazine suppressed the cholinergic system, and we have learned since that it also interacts with dopamine, an amine in the brain. Although dopamine is not directly involved in conscious-state control, it is crucial in mediating motivated behavior and it is a chemical cousin of norepinephrine. Thus the same general principle may unite our model of dream psychosis with Bertal's waking psychosis and its chemical management. Any condition (or drug) that alters the balance of the aminergic and cholinergic systems is likely to alter — for better or worse — brain-mind state.

THE BENEFITS OF DISTRACTION

In order to evaluate an attention-getting signal we need to free our brain-mind from its riveting control. The reflexive animal has a limited set of options; to be on the safe side, it usually just runs away. That may be safe, but it is neither economical nor supple. To be discriminating, we need immediate access to as large and rich a store of memory as possible, guided by experientially determined priorities. How do our brain-minds simultaneously accomplish the twin tasks of sharp focus and rich analysis? Let's circle back to our consideration of memory and emotion.

When we are awake, the aminergic system is dominant, but the cholinergic system still plays a role, which increases as the day wears on. And recall that, while the amines are necessary for recording an experience, it is acetylcholine that consolidates memory. In the dynamic struggle between the aminergic and cholinergic systems, we are witnessing a strategic trade-off between attentional selectivity (aminergic) and contextual versatility (cholinergic). This contrast fits well with our notion of foreground processing (of the constant flow of data from our immediate environment) and background processing (of plans, memories, and reference frames). It also fits well with the differences between waking and dreaming consciousness.

In sharply attentive awareness, when the aminergic system dominates brain-mind operations, the emphasis is on focus and response. In more relaxed waking, when the cholinergic system plays a more prominent role, a broader set of internal constructs (thoughts, memories, wishes, and desires) is used to reflect on ongoing events. In sleep, as both the aminergic and cholinergic systems abate, both focus and repertoire become sharply limited. In dreaming, focus is lost altogether as the aminergic system shuts off, but the response repertoire is correspondingly more vast because the cholinergic system is given unbridled sway.

This diurnal continuum of attention can be explained by the AIM model. In the morning our brain-minds are wide awake. Our attention is clear and sharp. We can focus — and we can switch — with relative ease. Our most successful colleagues can even keep several tasks on track at once. To do this, the aminergic system must be at its peak, and it has benefited from complete rest in REM sleep. We are in the waking segment, the upper, back, right-hand corner of the state space.

By afternoon or evening our attention is not so tightly connected to the external and internal information that competes for our consciousness. Our minds wander. We daydream. We are more easily distracted. Our fantasies shift from the dress-rehearsal, problem-solving mode of the morning, to more exotic, escapist, and sensual topics. We long for our families and friends, our lovers and our entertainment. This attentional transition corresponds to a gradual loss in aminergic power and a corresponding gain in the cholinergic ability to dilate, imagine, and freely associate. We have moved down toward the center of the state space.

Our daily glide down the curve is preparing us little by little for our nightly launch into the cholinergic world of our dreams. Logic is on hold, restoring itself, like norepinephrine, for the newspapers and spreadsheets of tomorrow. Once we have gone to bed and traveled the null zone of non-REM sleep, we switch to an uncritical and wild review of our memories and emotions. We pop the corks on our brain-mind stocks of acetylcholine and we are drawn down to the lower, front, right-hand corner of the state space. We indulge ourselves in dreaming. Our inattention favors our looking at everything, imaging things we never saw before. And as the versatility of our associative power is reassured, our attentional capacity is restored. We awaken.

CHAPTER 11

Ups and Downs: Energy, Mood, and Health

YOU CAN GET a whopping case of jet lag without ever leaving home. Just stay up all night and see what happens the next day. For even more fun, stay awake for a few nights running, sleep a bit during the days, and you will begin to experience some very peculiar shifts in your energy state and your conscious experience. Some are so dramatic they will put the effects of jet lag to shame. I've experienced this many times, after spending nights in the recording room of my sleep lab watching others sleep and monitoring their brain waves.

I discovered these shifts in energy for myself when I was doing all-night sleep studies at the National Institute of Mental Health in Bethesda, Maryland, early in my career. Night turned into my day, and evening turned into my morning. I would finish my experiments at about 7:00 A.M., make my rounds at the hospital, discuss the next night's experiment with my mentor, and drive back to Washington, D.C., to my apartment near the Washington Cathedral. I was so tired once I got there that, with the shades open, traffic roaring, and fire engines clanging, I could sleep without difficulty. By 10:00 A.M. I was out. I would set my alarm for 4:00 in the afternoon, so I could get up in time to greet my wife, Joan, when she got back from her teaching job at the Cathedral School.

In order to maintain our connection with the social world, we decided we would try to go out together in the evening as much as possible. Anyway, it was the early 1960s; we lived in JFK's Camelot Washington, and as young Bostonian transplants we were starry-eyed and eager to be in the swim. But it was frequently pointless. My body yelled, "Hell no! I won't go!"

My body said no because my brain-mind (that's me, after all) was in a morning mood, not an evening mood. It was ripe for a quiet breakfast and a leisurely read through the newspaper, and then primed for focused, analytical thinking. The boisterous, scattered energy of a cocktail party was not something my brain-mind could tolerate. I would look in stupefied disdain at the frenetic guests as if they were manic psychotics who needed lithium to bring them back down to the ground. They looked at me as if I were a depressive who needed electroshock therapy.

I wasn't depressed any more than they were manic. Our energy levels were simply out of phase with each other. The same thing happens after a long flight across several time zones; your energy, your body temperature, and your sleep rhythms don't beat in local time.

We all know that our energy oscillates between ups and downs. When we're up, the world is our oyster. We feel as if we can do anything. When we're down, all is bleak and dismal. Like Bertal, we may say to ourselves, "I should have stayed in bed." It seems clear, too, that when we are up we feel more healthy, and when we are down we feel our resistance to infection has fallen as low as our mood.

Can our knowledge about the brain-mind be extended beyond the brain-mind itself, to the body at large? Indeed it can, for the brain-mind closely regulates our energy, mood, and health. But how and why does our sleep schedule affect our energy level? Is good sleep required for good health? Are mental illnesses of energy and mood, such as depression, a function of brain-mind states? And can these illnesses be beaten by altering the states? The answer, as we will see, is that they most certainly can.

LINKING MIND TO BODY

The nervous system connects mind and body. On its broadest scale, our nervous system has two divisions — the central nervous system and the peripheral nervous system. The central nervous system consists of the brain and the spinal cord; it receives impulses from nerve fibers in the skin and organs and fires motor commands to muscles and glands. The peripheral nervous system consists of nerves that control the face, neck, and spine and the so-called autonomic nerves, which regulate the heart, lungs, stomach, and other organs.

The autonomic nervous system is the key to energy, mood, and health. It has two divisions of its own — the sympathetic nervous system and the parasympathetic nervous system. The sympathetic nervous system kicks our cardiovascular system into higher gear when we ask the heart and lungs to respond; its instructions are carried by amine molecules like norepinephrine. The parasympathetic nervous system slows the heart and lungs, using instructions carried by acetylcholine. Our understanding of the brain-mind can therefore be directly applied to the body for one significant reason: the division of labor between the aminergic and the cholinergic systems in our brains is mirrored by a division of labor between amines and acetylcholine in the body.

By asking our heart and lungs to increase their output, the sympathetic nervous system requires us to expend energy. Its action is described as ergotropic, which means energy generating. And by asking these organs to reduce their output, the parasympathetic nervous system tells us to conserve energy. Its action is described as trophotropic, which means energy conserving.

So, in a nutshell, here are the relationships we need to keep in mind:

Waking	*Sleeping*
amines	acetylcholine
ergotropic	trophotropic
sympathetic nervous system	parasympathetic nervous system
high energy output	low energy output

Now that we can speak the language of physiology, we can begin to determine why any of this matters. In both the brain and the body, all states that have high energy demands depend on the release of the amine norepinephrine from nerve cells. When norepinephrine rises after a night's sleep, we wake up. It remains high during waking and falls in defeat to acetylcholine when we go to sleep again. Since norepinephrine and acetylcholine regulate the major brain-mind states of waking and sleep, we see that energy flow must be an elemental aspect of these states. In its fundamental form, this idea strongly parallels the Eastern notion of yin and yang.

In the early half of this century, physiologists assumed that the autonomic nervous system was connected to and controlled by the brain, but they didn't know that the brain itself contained cholinergic neurons. When I went to medical school in the late 1950s, there was still no direct evidence that acetylcholine was a central brain neurotransmitter. Now we know that acetylcholine mediates REM sleep, during which energy is conserved. The reduced demand for output enables norepinephrine to be stockpiled against future energy demands.

Physiologists did know that acetylcholine slowed heart action. In fact the discovery of acetylcholine, by Otto Loewi, was made during research into heart-rate regulation, which can be a matter of life and death, for example, during cardiac arrest. It was speculated that when carried to extremes, the cholinergic system could so powerfully slow the heart that heartbeat would stop altogether, causing Voodoo Death. Although we've dropped the moniker, today's physiologists still believe that mediation of cardiac arrhythmia by acetylocholine can cause sudden death.

In the central parts of Thailand and Cambodia, there is a syndrome of sudden death in young men that occurs during sleep. As in other illnesses, death in sleep may be related to the normal tendency of acetylcholine to alter the rhythm of the heart, which is made abnormally sensitive by other physiological factors such as genetics or diet. Sleep death is called Lai Tai by the Thai natives, who believe it is caused by the vengeful visit of a widow ghost who seduces men in their dreams and kills them in retribution for their infidelity.

We can therefore conclude that the yin and yang of the brain and body are maintained by the reciprocity of the aminergic and cholinergic systems, which spring from nerve cells in the brain stem. The aminergic-cholinergic systems in the brain and body are also directly linked by the nerves in the brain stem, which guarantees the regular cycling we undergo from the energy-outputting waking state and the energy-conserving sleeping state.

While this sounds like common sense, it actually isn't. Common sense has always held that sleep conserved energy because it ensured inactivity and rest. After a good night's sleep we wake up feeling more alert and stronger. But sleep is commanded by the surge of the cholinergic system. Acetylcholine works at least as hard at night as it does during the day. Cholinergic brain cells are most active during REM sleep, and almost all the brain neurons are turned on. This discovery runs directly counter to common sense because it means that our mental refreshment must be achieved by a special kind of brain work, rather than brain rest. This shows us just how misleading subjective experience can be. We simply cannot intuit the way the brain functions from our psychology. We must have recourse to physiology.

REGULATING BODY TEMPERATURE

One energy function that is particularly sensitive to changes in brain-mind state is body temperature. Because it is so important it is appropriately called a "vital sign" by doctors, who record it every four hours when we are patients in a hospital. When body temperature rises or falls, we feel intensely uncomfortable and know that our health is threatened.

Mammals zealously maintain their body temperature within narrow limits. With the exception of the remarkable state of hibernation, body temperature in mammals normally fluctuates within the very small range of about 1.5°F. Body temperature typically peaks when we are awake and active, and dips when we are asleep and restful. The ergotropic-trophotropic energy cycle, which rises during waking and falls during sleep, determines the body's temperature curve. As it should; it costs more energy to keep our bodies warm when we are out and about than when we are lying still and covered in our beds.

Since our physiology is so dependent on tight regulation of temperature, it came as a great surprise to find that when mammals are in REM sleep, temperature control is essentially abandoned. This unexpected finding suggests that during REM sleep the brain's thermostat is temporarily turned off. The reason that body temperature does not fall during this time is because heat loss is prevented by sleep behavior. We sleep in warm nests or beds. And we don't sleep at all if we are cold. Explorers who are unexpectedly trapped overnight in frigid areas and don't have adequate protection try to stay awake; too many of their predecessors have fallen asleep under such conditions and frozen to death. Now we know why.

Temperature regulation depends on the activity of the sympathetic nervous system — the ergotropic system — which is modulated by norepinephrine. And we know what happens to the cells that produce norepinephrine during REM sleep: they are turned down to almost zero. So energy mobilization and temperature control are two tightly linked processes, and the link between them is provided by the aminergic system. When it is on, we are awake and our temperature is regulated. When it is off, we are in REM sleep and our temperature is not regulated.

When we are sick with the flu and our body reacts with fever, our sleep may become light and fitful. This occurs in part because the elevated temperature suppresses REM sleep and with it dreams, leaving our minds in the thrall of the persistent obsessive thinking of non-REM sleep and the microdreams of repeated and unsuccessful sleep onsets. However much we need to sleep, we have trouble getting enough of the right kind because our aminergic emergency defense system is too busy with survival to allow the luxury of deep cholinergic recuperation.

If REM sleep causes us to abandon temperature control, then why do our brain-minds ever allow our bodies to fall into such a precarious position? One idea is that REM sleep may function not only to conserve energy, but also to conserve the capacity to regulate energy flow properly. It is in REM sleep that we most effectively restore our aminergic system and therefore our ability to maintain a constant body temperature. Recall that we came to a similar conclusion about the aminergic-cholinergic system in the brain; the aminergic system is suspended during REM sleep so that it can restore itself and function properly when we most need it — when we are awake.

If REM sleep functions to rejuvenate the energy-regulation system, then sleep loss — over the long term — would have several potentially damaging results. One would be a loss of control over body temperature; another would be a loss of energy availability; and a third would be depression of brain-mind energy functions. We will see that, to a degree, all these outcomes have been shown in laboratory animal studies, and that ill health, depression, and even death may be the consequences of sleep loss. Recent experiments have revealed that long-term sleep loss invariably leads to death in rats and that the sleep-deprived rats die from infection.

SLEEP AND THE IMMUNE SYSTEM

None of the declarations of folk psychology is more widely believed than that linking good sleep and good health. Mothers have exhorted their children to "get a good night's sleep" since time began, it seems. In the early 1970s, studies conducted at the California Human Population Laboratory identified several behaviors that were positively correlated with length of life. Sleep headed the list, followed by exercise (which is known to promote sleep), eating breakfast (commuters take note), and not snacking (icebox raiders beware). Weight watching, not smoking, and moderating alcohol intake were also positive predictors of good health.

The subjects in the California study have been followed over time, and those with six of the seven health behaviors listed above have all enjoyed much longer lives than those who violated the rules. But longevity is not the only yardstick that measures the payoff. Positive well-being, or "feeling good," has been linked to all seven factors. It thus appears that not only life itself but wellness is somehow fostered by good sleep.

I say "somehow" to emphasize that the encouraging results of these epidemiological studies do not establish causality. For example, it could be that good sleep is not linked to good health at all, but that both are simply the effects of exercise. Or it could be that healthy people just happen to sleep well. It certainly seems that for us to have a sense of well-being, enjoyment, and accomplishment we need energy and a positive mood. And it seems natural that people who are depressed lack energy and have problems with mood. But we cannot feel secure in our well-being or help those who are depressed unless we can uncover the mechanisms that drive energy and mood. Is good health mediated by brain-mind states as they dictate the flow of norepinephrine, which controls waking the sympathetic nervous system, and acetylcholine, which controls sleep and the parasympathetic nervous system? Let's see what recent research tells us.

We all share a common experience when we have the flu; we feel best (or, should I say, least bad) in the morning, when we have "rested." Our symptoms worsen by afternoon and more so by evening. But we improve again after good sleep. Many people, including me, will swear by sleep for the flu until something better comes along. But can sleep actively suppress infection? Can it actually boost the immune system? That is exactly the conclusion reached by James Krueger of the University of Tennessee after fifteen years of research on the effects of sleep deprivation on rabbits, rats, mice, and — believe it or not — goats. Goats were chosen because they had proven useful in studies of cerebrospinal fluid, a rich source of some of the brain chemicals related to sleep.

To make a long and fascinating story short, it turns out that when animals are sleep deprived, a protein known as di-muramyl peptide accumulates in their spinal fluid. The peptides do not originate in the brain. Instead, they come from bacteria in the body, suggesting that sleep deprivation may enable bacterial growth and that sufficient sleep impedes bacterial growth.

What's even more interesting is that these di-muramyl peptides enhance non-REM sleep (but not REM sleep). The peptides also cause fever. The two effects are dissociable, however; the sleep effect is independent of the fever. More interesting still is the fact that the peptides stimulate cells in the brain and the body to produce interleukin-1, a powerful immune-system molecule that promotes the destruction of both bacteria and tumor cells. Highly significant and desirable health effects are mediated by interleukin's ability to encourage the B lymphocytes to produce antibodies, which kill viruses, and to trigger the proliferation of T lymphocytes, which attack microbial invaders. The net effect is to mobilize the body's defensive forces.

It looks as if sleep research has inadvertently stumbled on something of capital importance. By depriving his animals of sleep, Krueger made them more vulnerable to infection, which stimulated their immune system, which made them more sleepy. Having noticed this, it was then possible to show that many immune proteins do, in fact, promote sleep. Taking a shot of sleep for your flu is sounding better and better, isn't it? No needles. No pills. Sleep alone is enough to change the state of the immune system.

Now we return to our first question. Why do we feel sleepy when we have an infection? Perhaps because interleukin-1, a protein that is part of the normal bodily response to infection, is also an effective sedative. Like the peptides, interleukin-1 enhances non-REM sleep. It also increases the size of the EEG waves associated with non-REM sleep. Thus both the length and depth of sleep are increased as an integral part of the body's attempt to repulse microbial invaders. The upshot is that there is a positive, circular interaction between the immune response and sleep. Sleep enhances the immune system, and the immune system enhances sleep.

Invaders are assaulting our body's portals at all times, not just during winter, when we tend to get sick more, and not just during local outbreaks of viruses. This means that the margin of safety of our health — the degree to which we are resistant to infection, and perhaps even cancer — may be determined by how well our sleep state enhances our immune system. The daily sequencing of normal brain-mind states, therefore, mediates our health.

It is non-REM sleep that is enhanced by the chemicals our bodies produce to fight infection. Why is REM sleep absent from the immune response picture? We're not sure, but it seems likely it is because REM sleep involves a loss of temperature control. When we are sick, our body temperature soars and drops, and we cannot risk entering REM sleep and abandoning temperature control.

REM AS SUPERSLEEP

We have seen how non-REM sleep helps us battle infection. Once we are healthy, however, it seems that REM sleep is the key to staying on top of our game. We have noted thus far that REM sleep serves to restore our energy system. Recall, too, from our discussion of memory, that during REM sleep our memory is consolidated and made permanent. During this unique brain-mind state of REM sleep, then, our circuits are being cleared and our battery is being recharged. We wake up with the insight and energy needed to tackle problems that seemed insoluble the night before.

As the conservator of the aminergic system, REM sleep is more than twice as effective as non-REM sleep. The firing rates of neurons containing norepinephrine and serotonin drop to half their waking levels in non-REM sleep, but the output drops by far more than half again in REM sleep. Thus REM sleep is at least five times more conservative of the amines than non-REM sleep and ten times more conservative than waking.

These calculations are based on the assumptions that the release of the chemical modulators is directly proportional to the firing rate of the neurons and that there is no release when the cells don't fire at all. Both assumptions have not been proven directly, but the general conclusion that far fewer amines are released in REM sleep than in either non-REM sleep or waking *has* been proven by experiments that measure their concentration in the brain. The same methods have also shown reciprocal increases in acetylcholine.

REM, it seems, is some sort of supersleep. The first reason for according it this status is that, although it normally occupies only about 20 percent of the total time we sleep each night, it takes only six weeks of deprivation of REM sleep alone to kill rats compared with four weeks for complete sleep deprivation. Based on its relative duration of only 20 percent of sleep time, we would predict that five times as long a deprivation period would be required if both states were equally life-enhancing. On these terms, one minute of REM sleep is worth five minutes of non-REM sleep.

The second reason supporting the idea of REM as supersleep is one that is attractive for the nappers of the world: there is a surprisingly beneficial nature of short naps if they occur at times in the day when REM sleep probability is high. Daytime naps are different from night sleep in that we may fall directly into a REM period and stay there for the duration of the nap. Since the time of peak REM probability is greatest in the late morning, the tendency of naps to be composed of REM sleep is highest then and falls thereafter till the onset of night sleep (about twelve hours later). The implication is that a little bit of sleep, at the right time of day, may be more useful than the same amount later on.

The third reason is that, following the deprivation of even small amounts of REM sleep, there is a prompt and complete repayment. The subject who has been denied REM sleep launches into extended REM periods as soon as he is allowed to sleep normally. In recent drug studies, when REM sleep was prevented the payback seemed to be made with interest. More REM sleep was paid back than was lost.

Of course, all these considerations have ignored the prospect that we might derive benefits from the rise of acetylcholine during REM sleep too. Unfortunately, how acetylcholine might confer its positive trophotropic benefits is as yet obscure. One possibility is that exposure to high levels of acetylcholine might affect cell metabolism. If so, this would indicate a link between brain-mind states and genetics, an exciting scientific prospect.

The field of brain-mind research is on the threshold of an inevitable union with molecular biology. Since both REM sleep and DNA were discovered in 1953, this is a rather late marriage. The neuromodulator molecules — norepinephrine, serotonin, and acetylcholine — operate on the membrane surface of cells. Genes are large molecules that lie deep in the nucleus of the cell. Genes communicate via messenger molecules that ferry information from cell membranes to the nucleus. There is evidence that the neuromodulators may affect this communication. If this is the case, then norepinephrine, serotonin, and acetylcholine may affect the communication between genes. And since they affect the brain-mind states, they would provide a link between our genes and our states.

Thus we can contemplate a very intimate conjunction in biology: the coupling of sleep to our genes. From such a union the fathers of DNA and REM sleep, Francis Crick, James Watson, Eugene Aserinsky, and Nathaniel Kleitman, could expect a bevy of beautiful scientific grandchildren.

My hypothesis, and that of many sleep scientists, is that each of the three major brain-mind states — waking, sleeping, and dreaming — will prove to be quite different states at a very deep level, that of gene expression. Genes operate by making enzymes, and enzymes are essential to synthesizing norepinephrine, serotonin, and acetylcholine. We might expect, then, that in REM sleep the genetic manufacture of enzymes that synthesize the norepinephrine molecule would be turned on when acetylcholine interacts with the messenger cells communicating with the genes. A related concept would be that the disappearance of norepinephrine during REM sleep might signal genes to crank out more of the enzymes that make it. Either way, by the time we wake up enough norepinephrine will have been manufactured so that the aminergic system is ready to go. What scientists need, now, are ways to study the genetic biology of sleep. As genetics and brain-mind theory come together, we will find better explanations of how states affect energy, mood, and health.

THE STATE OF DEPRESSION

Meanwhile, we are making great progress in understanding some mental illnesses that would seem to be directly linked to energy level. People who are depressed, for example, sleep poorly and often complain of feeling tired. They want to sleep all the time, yet their sleep does not rejuvenate them. Their bodies feel "heavy," and alertness is replaced by a kind of dazed semi-consciousness. Exercise, which most patients with depression know would help break the force of this vicious downward spiral, is not initiated because people suffering from depression don't feel like exercising. They can't get up enough energy to do it in the first place. The trophotropic system seems to act without opposition, pulling these people down, down, down into the slough of despondency and lethargy. Food becomes unappealing, so energy supplies decrease further. Weight loss then occurs. Sexual energy and libido are gone. These people are on their way to a vegetative death.

What is going on in the state-control centers of the brain stem during depression? How are the brain-mind states affected? And how can the vicious cycle be reversed?

People who suffer from depression exhibit two significant shifts in sleep rhythm: one affects the timing of rest and activity across a twenty-four-hour day; the other affects the timing of the first REM period during sleep. Both may have a common cause — the lowered efficacy of the aminergic system, which revs up the brain during waking and mediates the storm of acetylcholine release during sleeping. People who are depressed are directly experiencing low ebbs of chemical power in their brains and bodies.

The first problem, that of the timing of sleep and waking, arises because our natural sleep-wake cycle is not twenty-four hours. Scientists know this by studying people who are isolated from time cues; experiments performed on people who are sequestered in underground bunkers show that our natural cycle is from 24.3 to 25.0 hours. Therefore, if left to our own devices, we would go to sleep a bit later every night and wake up a bit later every morning.

We don't follow this sleep phase delay, though, because our brain-minds use social cues, clocks, adherence to work hours, and such to reset our sleep cycle via our behavior so that it falls into a twenty-four-hour phase. Our physiology has helped us adapt also; the internal clock that controls our daily cycle is in the hypothalamus, just above the pituitary gland. It is located just behind the crossing point of the two eye nerves. The eye nerves send fibers directly into the hypothalamus. Scientists assume these fibers convey information about day length to help the brain clock reset itself each day.

The proper care and management of our brain-mind states thus involves the rewinding of our brain clocks. People who succumb to depression fail to reset their clocks properly. It has been shown that use of artificial light, and even sleep deprivation, can have beneficial effects on depressed mood, by helping the brain and body get themselves back into phase.

The second problem for depressives is the timing of REM sleep. Ironically, even though depressives are always tired and always want to sleep, more sleep is their own worst enemy. REM sleep makes depression worse, and REM deprivation makes depression better. How can this be?

Depressed subjects who are studied in the sleep lab exhibit two unusual characteristics. First, they are unlikely to have any deep non-REM sleep. Although we are not sure why this is so, the outcome suggests that the depth of sleep is lessened, accounting for its unrefreshing quality. So more non-REM sleep will not help the depressive.

The second odd characteristic is that the first REM sleep period occurs earlier, lasts longer, and is more intense than usual. It is as if the process that normally restrains REM sleep is weakened, while the process that normally drives it is intensified. REM sleep is normally restrained by norepinephrine and serotonin; although they are down, they are not out during dreaming and put at least some rein on the cholinergic system that causes REM sleep. It is no surprise, though, that the strength of the aminergic system would be diminished in depression. The cause of energy loss in the body results from a depressed sympathetic nervous system, that is, a depressed aminergic system. A parallel weakness appears in the brain's aminergic system. The body and the brain-mind suffer from aminergic inefficacy. Failure of the aminergic system could be due to several things: the brain stem isn't making enough norepinephrine or serotonin; or the brain stem is not delivering the chemicals fast enough to their targets; or those targets are not receptive to the chemicals when they arrive.

This reduced ability to receive the amines may be a consequence of anxiety. Anxiety causes excessive transmission of amines, which demands excessive reception of amines. Over time, our cells simply can't keep up; their ability to continually accept amines becomes exhausted.

Whatever the cause, we need to give the aminergic system a jump start. It needs a jolt so that it will kick over and squirt out some of that high-energy juice. Perhaps that's why the treatment of depression by electroshock is sometimes so effective, or why a good game of squash or a good aerobic workout helps us feel "up." When we exercise, we force our aminergic system to increase output; more norepinephrine is needed to rev up our heart rate and breathing. A parallel heightening of norepinephrine occurs in the brain. With regular exercise, the aminergic system becomes more robust and is better able to control REM sleep, bringing the depressive back into the proper sleep cycle and slowly lifting him out of the abyss. Jolting of the aminergic system by stimulant drugs is almost certainly the reason that they work too; they mimic the action of norepinephrine and energize us. They aren't called "uppers" for nothing.

Could REM sleep deprivation be another way of strengthening the neurons that produce amines? At first glance, it may seem so. Preventing REM sleep would depress the cholinergic system, allowing the aminergic system to gain back some ground. But this will never work for the long term because tension will build up in the cholinergic system, and at some point it will overtake the brain-mind in a dangerous way. Remember, that's what caused me to hallucinate my sudden helper at the woodshed. And remember that REM sleep deprivation in lab animals leads to death. That's all too definitive a cure!

How about more REM sleep, say, by napping? No help. Depressed people who nap wake up even worse than they were before. Weird. Shouldn't they have saved some energy if REM sleep is supersleep? No, because the depressed person's system is already hypersensitive to acetylcholine. The last thing a depressive's brain cells need is a rising flood of acetylcholine during REM sleep.

We can test this in the lab with a cholinergic drug called arecoline. When administered to a normal person who is sleeping, it triggers a dream epoch during non-REM sleep. This "cholinergic dreaming" is an altered brain-mind state caused by deliberate chemical intervention. It might be, then, that by using this drug to trigger dreaming during non-REM, a depressive's aminergic system could recuperate during these epochs. But the plan backfires because the induced REM sleep turns on the person's cholinergic brain cells, which produce more acetylcholine, to which they are

already hypersensitive. Here the vicious cycle of depression reveals
itself at the cellular-molecular level.

ANTIDEPRESSANT DRUGS

Something more definitive must occur if a rise in the power of
the aminergic system is to be sustained. Recent discoveries indicate
the place to look is within our own DNA — our genes. This may
be a clue as to how the antidepressant drugs really work and why
they often take so long to pep patients up.

Until we find the exact mechanism, people who suffer from depression can take solace in knowing that antidepressant drugs do
work. All the drugs of the now legion class of antidepressants have
the desirable property of increasing the power of the aminergic
brain cells.

Many of the antidepressants are not only pro-aminergic but also
anti-cholinergic. They interfere with the ability of cells to produce
acetylcholine, which is desirable because the depressive person is
hypersensitive to acetylcholine. This aid is not without a bad side,
though. Acetylcholine mediates many mechanisms in the brain and
body, and the drugs are not selective. They act everywhere in the
body that acetylcholine acts. This causes many side effects, such as
dry mouth and fainting. So in the long run knowing the specific,
cellular mechanism of depression will serve us well.

Immediately, when a depressed person starts to take one of
these drugs, his distinctive sleep abnormalities are reversed. But the
changes in brain-cell chemistry do not immediately and directly
alter mood. Some later, longer-term process is involved.

To picture this long-term process, consider the time it takes for
a country to mobilize defense forces. When war is declared, the
citizens are in alarm. They immediately initiate strategies like running the munitions factories twenty-four hours a day and converting chemical plants from the manufacture of nitrate fertilizer
to the making of nitroglycerine. We turn plowshares into swords,
but it may take months, or years, to reach peak production. In the
brain, it takes two to three weeks.

RESTORING ENERGY, MOOD, AND HEALTH

Sleep and the antidepressant drugs both appear to be keys to the same locks. The way sleep beats the flu may have much in common with the way that antidepressants alter mood. The brain and the immune system are homologous in requiring an appreciable time to mobilize the forces that give us energy, health, and our sense of well-being.

In the case of the immune system, it is not hard for us to imagine why it takes some time to defeat a microbial invader. The antibody factory has to be turned on and must produce enough molecules to slow the growth of the rapidly multiplying bacteria or virus. In the time it takes to get the defense system moving the infectious agents may not only be proliferating but digging in and — like an invading army — making themselves more difficult to dislodge. Infections, like wars, can go on and on.

People who are depressed are often not only low in energy but so stuck in their thoughts that they can't get going in any direction. Their ideas become so black and their outlook so bleak that they don't even see the point of trying to get going, or consulting a doctor, or taking the pills he may prescribe. And just as they do not usually fall into the slough of despondency overnight, they rarely pull out of it in a day. These long-term effects, I propose, can work only by changing the metabolism of our brain cells. These cells are slow to fall and slow to rise again even when pushed by the helping hand of a drug. I will return to this topic in Part Three.

DELIA AND BERTAL

Depression is a disorder of energy. The first step toward depression, a general feeling of being down, may be brought on by a number of causes. It can arise due to a sense of loss following anything from death of a loved one to bankruptcy. It can also be brought on by anxiety. People who allow themselves to be overcome with anxiety start to feel they are trapped, they can't win; they are already sliding down the slippery slope into depression.

Their mind says, "I can't do it," and their body says, "I have no energy for it." There is a parallel psychological and physiological response. This is no surprise, since the aminergic systems of the brain and body are linked.

If this is true, and the underlying premise of this book — that normal and abnormal states are variants of the same thing — holds, then a similar trigger for depression should cause similar symptoms in someone who is emotionally stable and someone who is psychotic. We have two ready subjects to compare: Delia and Bertal.

During the time Delia was keeping her journal, there were days when she, like everyone else, did appear to be anxious. After I got to know her a bit better, it became clear that her own anxiety was related in part to living alone. Generally, Delia could handle this anxiety. But once in a while, when she was starkly reminded of her difficulties, she would feel so downtrodden that she wanted to stay in bed instead of getting up and going to work.

This localized depression — the psychological feeling of being down and the physical feeling of being tired — appeared not only in her waking state but in her dreaming state as well. This indicates that although dream emotion has a consistent profile that is widely shared by most people, there still might be important shifts in that profile as individuals undergo life stress. In the case of the loss of a loved one, for example, we might expect both the dream content and the dream emotion to reflect our pain.

DELIA'S "ANIMATION" DREAM

I was watching what I took to be a piece of animation. The viewpoint of the observer was floating into an elaborate watergarden-like scene of trees, sky, and still water. The piece impressed me because it was all apparently done with watercolors, a difficult medium, and since the viewpoint was sweeping into the piece, no loops could be used in animating the sequence — each panel had to have been painted separately. This would have meant an immense amount of work to produce even a short piece.

The scene shifted to a scene of an old-world city street, like an alleyway, surrounded by the brick walls of buildings and with people walking on the sidewalks. Again, I was amazed by the detail. The people looked real, but I knew the scene was not real and I couldn't figure out how it was done. It looked like it might have been done with still motion photography. I slapped a brick wall and popped my lips with my hand to see if the sound coincided with the scenery. It did. I decided it must have been done with computer animation.

The dream again shifted, this time into an opera performed by my father and mother. Another man was trying to steal my mother away. My father intervened to take my mother back, but my mother ran back to the other man. My father then pulled her away and looked like he might hit her. At that point I intervened myself to prevent this. My father stomped off to a men's room and my mother escaped to a lady's room. I commented to Larry, who was there and with whom I was going to see a movie, that no matter what everyone was saying (since the opera was in another language) the action had put me in a foul mood.

The day following the dream, Delia was very depressed, not only because of the dream, but also because mentally and physically she felt defeated. Feelings of anxiety had mounted to a point that they triggered a psychotic event — a dream about her parents' marriage. And after the dream, Delia felt more depressed than before it.

This is exactly the same pattern Bertal experienced. His mother brought him to The Psycho a short time after he had received a promotion at his electronics job. He couldn't handle the increased responsibility. He felt like a failure, and his self-esteem plummeted. The anxiety built inside him. During the two weeks prior to the day his mother convinced him to get into the car (so she could drive him to The Psycho), he had withdrawn more and more from houseguests, his siblings, and even his mother. He ate poorly and began to lose weight. Once he got to The Psycho he became still more anxious and began to have psychotic episodes — hallucinations. After each episode, he was intractable. Remember when I found him on the kitchen floor after a hallucination? He stayed there motionless for an hour; he could not move even if he had wanted to.

When he was at the height of his panic, he spoke only in short, cryptic phrases, indicating a strong preoccupation with sex and violence, such as the following:

"S.O.S."

"Theresa is having a baby."

"Communists."

"Shock treatment destroys the brain."

"Violence destroys the body."

"Kotex."

Following that scene he was severely depressed for several days; he stayed in bed much of the time, did not come to his scheduled sessions with me, and ate little.

Bertal's symptoms were much more extreme than Delia's, but they arose from the same psychological source, followed the same sequence, and had the same effects on mind and body. And neither Delia nor Bertal, in these instances, got out of the depression until they got out of their beds and got back into their routines, which raised new — but manageable and familiar — challenges that got their aminergic systems going again.

We now know that jump-starting our energy systems can often be achieved more easily by giving the aminergic system a chemical kick. In the last chapter of this book I will examine the pros and cons of exercising this option. Although there are some problems associated with any drug, the new antidepressants are particularly attractive because they do increase the power of the brain's aminergic energy system.

CHAPTER 12

What Is Consciousness?
What Is the Mind?

IN PART ONE, I described the basic chemistry of the brain (the aminergic-cholinergic system) and defined three of the forces (activation energy, information source, and modulation) that dictate the state we are in at every moment of our lives. Our many brain-mind states are controlled by these variables, and as the variables change, our brain-minds move from one state to another.

In the last six chapters I have shown that the major faculties we possess as human beings depend on the state of the brain-mind. When we are awake, "perception" means one thing; when we are asleep — or psychotic or daydreaming or panicked — perception means something quite different.

Now that it is possible to describe how our states are generated and how they affect all that we experience, I propose to answer two of the most fundamental questions in psychology and neurology: What is consciousness? And what is the mind?

If my sense of identity, location, and time (orientation), my representations of the world (perception), my stories and beliefs about my life (memory), my emotional states and inclinations (emotion and instinct), my capacity to direct my perceptions and thoughts (attention), and my well-being and zest for life (energy) all arise from brain-mind states, then I posit two theorems: (1) The mind is all the information in the brain. (2) Consciousness is the brain's awareness of some of that information.

A NEW DEFINITION OF CONSCIOUSNESS

On the face of it, these two statements may seem innocuous enough. But if you think about them closely, you will see that I probably have just discarded your very sense of who you are, and I have certainly forsaken the definitions of mind and consciousness used by most psychologists, psychiatrists, neurologists, and philosophers. For one thing, it appears that I have put the cart before the horse.

Most people, and most scientists, share a common notion that the mind springs from consciousness. When we sleep, we say our minds are at rest since our consciousness has been "turned off." We say someone who is psychotic is "out of his mind," meaning that he has lost an awareness of himself and the world around him.

We even go so far as to believe that there is a "seat of consciousness" in our brains somewhere. This idea goes way back to René Descartes. He designated the pineal gland as the seat of awareness, the seat of the soul, because of its budlike structure and its position in the middle brain. We would be equally mistaken today if we designated the pons as the seat of consciousness because it regulates the chemistry that controls our brain-mind states. Consciousness cannot be localized in any part of the brain, not even the cortex. It is distributed in many parts of the brain — and beyond.

Why does this seem to offend us? Is it any less satisfying to say that consciousness is everywhere in our brain-minds and even in our bodies? If we brush against a hot stove, our nerve endings send messages that indicate, "Wow, that's hot; better stay away from it." And if our hand happens to touch the burner, it is jerked away by a reflex action that bypasses the brain altogether. In both cases, we are aware of the world and are reacting to it. Is this not consciousness? I say emphatically, yes! Although my sensory nerves are not, themselves, capable of representing the world, the interconnected cells that receive their sensory messages are. The activation state of even these lowly nerve fibers is an essential component of my consciousness. The level and kind of consciousness that any brain-mind will have is a function of the number of neurons it possesses, the number of interconnections between them, the level of computation that they can support, and the nature of the states during which these computations take place.

Within any given individual, like me or you or Delia or Bertal, consciousness varies, continuously and gradually, through an infinite range of levels — from coma to enlightenment, from psychosis to poetry, from open suggestibility to rigid bigotry — as the simple result of the processing that is going on in our brains and the data that is being outwardly sensed and tapped from within. With this view, we can begin to consider how consciousness develops within members of a species and across species. When my daughter Julia was a baby, she could feel rage as part of a primordial conscious state long before she could name, tame, or explain it. Both my dog and cat can feel shame and can recognize me as their friend, without knowing what shame is or that I am an entity known as a person.

Allowing that consciousness develops gradually within and across creatures has the great advantage of freeing the concept from the straitjacket of language, in which it has often been corseted. To be sure, language does confer a special quality to the consciousness of those creatures who can speak, because their internal representations, as well as their communications with others, can be both propositional and abstract. For humans, possessing language thrusts consciousness up to such a level of richness, complexity, and inventiveness that it has prompted us to draw a self-congratulatory line between our own species and all others. But I defy you to find a single pet owner who would say his animal friend is devoid of consciousness or even a conscience. Furthermore, he would certainly say his pet is sometimes happy and other times sad. The line between us and "the rest of the animal world" has been sharply drawn only because it reinforces the dogmatic view of the uniqueness of humanity and its place in the grand scheme of things.

This view is flawed, not to mention conceited. Consciousness varies with each state, within a species, and between species. And as we have seen, the brain is never "turned off" or even resting; it is processing information all the time.

A NEW DEFINITION OF THE MIND

If consciousness is the brain's awareness of some of its information, then what is the mind? It is simply all the information in the brain. In this definition, mind is more fundamental than consciousness because most of the information that is in the brain at any point in time is not conscious. We cannot sense the programs that tell us how to breathe, when to sleep, how to remember, and even how to think. It all just happens. The best we can do is figure out how to use these capabilities to our advantage.

This will be a sticky place for many readers. It is hard to accept that "the mind" includes such basic activity as the routine firing of neurons that keeps us breathing. But I hope to convince you that by accepting the modest proposal that the mind includes nonconscious brain activity, you will gain important intellectual freedom and power at the cost of only hubris and self-glorification.

Broadening the definition of mind to include the genetically determined information that is in the brain, as well as that which is acquired or "learned," will also strike many readers as not only degrading but downright dangerous. Doesn't this make the word "mind" almost meaningless, since practically everything about the brain is, in a sense, stored information? In this view, the word "mental" also seems to be downgraded. We consider ourselves mental and other animals not. We equate mental function with thinking, but inside the brain, performing a math exercise or arguing over Freud is no different from keeping the heart going. In each operation, neurons are communicating with other neurons in exactly the same way; they are just different neurons firing in different places in the brain.

What we are after here is a more accurate and useful view of the concept of the mind than the one afforded by the anthropocentric view that mind entails consciousness, and that consciousness, in turn, entails language.

Suppose a snail learns to associate a shock stimulus to its tail with a painful prick to its snout. In time it will withdraw its snout when its tail is shocked whether or not its snout is subsequently pricked. This is classical conditioning, the fundamental paradigm of learning, and it has proven immensely useful in our efforts to understand the cellular and molecular basis of how our own thoughts, feelings, and actions are shaped by experience. So do you say that this is not mental activity because snails don't have consciousness and therefore they don't have minds? Or do you say that any learning is mental because it changes the status of information in the snail's brain? Mentality is the processing of information, whether or not it is done consciously.

Let's reconsider Delia's dreams. Dreaming is a conscious state of Delia's brain-mind, despite the fact that she does not experience it in the same way she would if awake. This means there is a continuity of the mind in the absence of waking consciousness; the people, plots, and emotions of Delia's dreams carry over directly from the people, plots, and emotions in her waking life. Her mind — the same mind that operates when she is awake — is operating when she is dreaming.

And when did Delia start experiencing this brain-mind state called dreaming? Did she begin to have dreams before she learned to speak or only after her speech had developed? In other words, do babies have minds? Almost everyone would say yes, they do, even though it is impossible to know for certain whether or not they are conscious in any way that resembles the adult sense of the word. And they certainly don't have language at their disposal. When, then, did Delia's mental life really begin? Did Delia already have a mind and some sort of dream experience before she was born? We know she had lots of REM sleep when she was floating in her mother's uterus. When did Delia's dreaming begin? Can we draw a sharp line? I don't think so.

As with the snail, the question becomes this: At what level of brain development do we say "the mind begins *now*." There is none. The mind is nothing but the information in the brain, and dreaming is nothing but the activation of that information. As such, all brain activation is deeply and essentially mental.

I am quite aware of the potential for abuse that this line of reasoning offers to those who hold that abortion should be banned because the human mind begins at the moment of conception. To them I would say that such decisions must be left to prospective parents without regard to the scientifically unresolvable issue of when consciousness or mind begins. We can *never* say conclusively. Furthermore, at no point in my theory is there any place for a separate entity, whether it be called mind or soul, that could either antedate or survive the brain. Whatever mind or soul there is, it is born, lives, and dies with the brain. In fact, there are cases when the mind dies while the brain is still alive, but is no longer capable of self-activation. Technically and legally, we refer to this permanent state of inactivation as "brain death."

CONSCIOUS AND NONCONSCIOUS

I have said that consciousness is the brain-mind's awareness of some of its own information. This bears further explanation. But first let me be clear on terminology. Much of the confusion about what consciousness is (or isn't) and about what mental activity is (or isn't) stems from the welter of contradictory terms used to describe the supposed strata of the mind.

We have all heard of the conscious, the subconscious, the unconscious, the nonconscious, the preconscious, the repressed unconscious, and so on. What a mess! All we need are two terms: conscious and nonconscious.

Historically, psychologists and writers have referred to the unconscious and subconscious minds as synonymous yet different. "Subconscious" is taken to mean just below conscious, while unconscious implies a negative, that is, no consciousness. Sure, if you're hit over the head with a brick you'll fall to the ground and be unconscious. As a medical term this has some usefulness, but that is all. Freud complicated matters further by dividing the un- or sub-conscious into a segment that has access to consciousness (the "preconscious") and one that does not (the "dynamically re-pressed unconscious"). Freud based his whole theory of mental life, including dreams and psychosis, on this conception. All these categories are just that — artificial constructs.

Given the monumental size of our current ignorance of these matters, it seems wisest to note simply that most of the information in the brain is nonconscious and to keep an open mind about what data can be admitted or excluded from consciousness. It also seems wisest for a simple and obvious reason: if our mind is all the information in our brain, then the information is either accessible (conscious) or inaccessible (nonconscious). It cannot exist in any other mode.

This is not a rigid segmentation. Data can move from one mode to the other. Remember my long-lost childhood friend Dick Tinguely, who popped into my dream one night after a fifty-two-year absence from my thoughts? He was buried in my nonconscious mind all that time, yet one night crossed over into consciousness. All our thoughts and willed actions are conscious. The motor programs that control our thinking and moving are nonconscious. And yet, people who are supposedly paralyzed sometimes, somehow, can begin to get movement back by sheer will. People who put themselves into a deep trance can sometimes, somehow, slow their own heartbeats. We "cross the line" ourselves in less mysterious but no less impressive ways every day, when we daydream and when we have our nightly REM-sleep dreams.

A corollary, bold but simple, is that all the information in the brain, whether conscious or nonconscious, is mental in that it can serve to solve the organism's adaptive problems and aid in achieving the two life goals of survival and procreation.

The information that can move from the nonconscious into consciousness includes much of what we call memory. Memory consists of perceptions that we can call forth as imagery, most of our emotions, most of our instincts, and a vast set of procedural talents. Many of the brain processes that are required to represent these kinds of data are themselves below the reach of consciousness. I propose calling the aggregate of these brain information states the nonconscious mind. We cannot intuitively know our nonconscious minds. Only observation, inference, and experiment help us realize its existence.

The division of mind into conscious and nonconscious components has many important advantages over the outmoded but still popular model of psychoanalysis. The most important advantage and difference of the new model is that it accomplishes precisely what Freud wanted to achieve when he set out, in 1890, to create a scientific psychology, a project that he later abandoned. Instead of creating a burden by insisting that a hidden cause for dreams, hallucinations, and delusions exists in some interaction between supposed layers of the mind, the new model offers a simple explanation: the imagery and emotions of dreams are always with us, riding in our nonconscious, and when we change state from waking to dreaming this information is able to cross into consciousness. Our dreams are not mysterious phenomena, they are conscious events. Here's the simplest test: Are we aware of what happens in our dreams? Of course. Therefore, dreaming is a conscious experience.

Note that the brain-mind offers a mechanism for this free flow of information; its continuously changing states enable information to flow from nonconscious to conscious. The phenomenon is inextricably tied to brain process. What happens with information in the conscious and nonconscious compartments of the mind depends on the state of the brain.

Thus I strongly agree with Freud's assertion that all mental data and all psychological concepts must ultimately find their roots in the physics and chemistry of the brain. Too many professional caretakers today hide behind the hocus-pocus of confused terminology and unprovable assertions in justifying the high rates they charge their patients or the unfounded theories they use to obtain grant money.

These folks will prove fatal to psychology. As scientific fact replaces psychological conjecture, they are hiding behind a new shield called hermeneutics — the study of texts. Rather than prove their assertions and diagnoses, they are now asserting that they never claimed to be scientific, that they were only studying the texts of Freud, or studying the utterings of psychotics, and interpreting them, as if this in some predictable way would result in help to those people with mental illnesses. It is both logically unjustified and ethically wrong to argue that hermeneutics can proceed independent of testing or proof by any other means. It is also wrong when people who purport to be helping the ill purely by studying texts — mostly religious scholars, university professors, and psychologists — claim to possess some sort of higher knowledge that is above or beyond experimental verification. Our new model of conscious and nonconscious is entirely compatible with the burgeoning sciences of the brain (neurobiology), the mind (cognitive science), and the integration of the two (cognitive neuroscience). It can be tested, and it can be verified.

IS THE MIND CAUSAL?

It is important to test our new view of the mind against a fundamental requirement of science and philosophy: causality. No explanation of the physical or metaphysical world passes muster if it cannot be explained in terms of cause and effect. As Sir Isaac Newton found out the hard way, apples fall from trees because of gravity. Gravity exists because masses attract each other. Masses attract each other because of forces between protons, neutrons, and electrons. And so it goes.

In our new view of the mind, causality is guaranteed. This is so because the workings of the brain-mind are rooted in the laws of physics and chemistry, which are themselves causal. A rise of the amines causes waking; being awake for the entire day weakens the amines, which enables acetylcholine to surge; this brings on non-REM sleep, which causes amines to drop lower and acetylcholine to rise so high that dreaming occurs; this enables the amines to rest and regroup, which causes waking again. Likewise, waking enables us to accept new information into our conscious minds, sleeping enables us to etch this information into the permanent memories of our nonconscious minds, and REM dreaming and daydreaming and other changes in state enable that information to travel between the two modes.

A bolder view, which some would debate, is that the REM-sleep state can initiate upward causation from the nonconscious to the conscious mind. In other words, an event at the nonconscious level — the firing of cholinergic neurons — could be said to cause the visions of our dreams.

As a corollary, dream forgetting is caused by the unavailability of norepinephrine and serotonin to the cells of the brain that store recent memories.

The boldest and most difficult argument to sustain is that there is downward causation from the conscious to the nonconscious mind — lucid dreaming, for example. Suppose I want to notice my dreams. To do so, I prime my brain-mind, before I go to sleep, to recognize later during REM that I am dreaming. This takes some persistence, but it usually works. Suppose I now decide to wake up from a dream. I can do so by an effort of will. This means that my conscious intent, instantiated as a specific chemical process, has actually caused the REM state to abate so that I can awaken with sharp and extensive recall of my dream.

REALIGNING PSYCHOLOGY AND NEUROLOGY

If we cannot, except under the most unusual circumstances, willingly access our own nonconscious mind, then how can it be studied? The best we can do is to objectively and experimentally study the nonconscious mind in other subjects and apply the findings to ourselves. There is no way for me to intuit directly the neuronal activation patterns of my brain stem. I can construct a model only by observing the activity of neurons in some other brain and hypothesize that my brain obeys the same rules. I imagine that I too possess a brain stem. I assume that my brain stem contains aminergic neurons that stop firing in REM sleep. I further assume that when my cholinergic neurons become enthusiastically active they spritz my thalamus with jets of acetylcholine and I dream. But even the articulation of such clear and specific ideas cannot lead me to directly perceive their reality. I can perceive only their effects on my own conscious states.

The nonconscious mind is forever closed to investigation via introspection. This principle casts further light on the folly of the Freudian enterprise. Freud believed that the "unconscious" could be investigated via introspection. With the assistance of a psycho-analyst versed in the method of free association, a person could trace the origins of bizarre dream content back to repressed instinc-tual wishes. Freud concocted a wild panoply of far-fetched expla-nations, most of them sexual, for dream stimuli, when we know today that dreams rise out of simple brain chemistry. When Freud said that dreaming was the "royal road to the unconscious," he failed to recognize that only a very small part of what actually determines dreaming is ever accessible to consciousness. To make his program work he was therefore obliged to bend his interpreta-tive scheme to the breaking point. As I pointed out in detail in my first book, *The Dreaming Brain,* practically every aspect of dream-ing is more clearly, more economically, and more profoundly un-derstood by passing the detour to Freud's royal road and taking the main avenue to the nonconscious mind afforded by neurobiology.

An important implication of this argument is that conscious-ness, however elegant and elevated a phenomenon it may be, is extremely limited in understanding itself. Scientists have repeatedly pointed out how misleading — and therefore unreliable — intro-spection can be. If we accept this, we can learn to use it better for the few things it can do well — such as describe the subjective as-pects of our brain-mind states — without forcing it to explain ev-ery facet of our lives.

The brain-mind paradigm thus unburdens consciousness from a responsibility it can never meet. It brings aid in the form of chem-ical explanations that can be tested and verified with the investiga-tive tools of modern technology. In doing so it shows why not only psychoanalysis, but all of speculative philosophy, is severely limited in what it can hope to understand about the mind. The mind is not only elusive by virtue of its being hidden from itself, it is literally embodied in the depths of brain cells and brain-mind states that cannot be illuminated by introspection.

This limitation is exactly why modern analytical philosophers, led by Bertrand Russell and Alfred North Whitehead, have talked themselves out of almost all claims regarding the mind and have settled instead for the logic of mathematics. It is also the reason psychoanalysts have increasingly restricted themselves to hermeneutics. Although these strategic retreats may be intellectually interesting, they are disappointing to people living in the real world, because it seems to us as if the analytical philosophers and psychoanalysts have abandoned the very purpose their disciplines were created to serve: to understand how the mind works in health and how it malfunctions in disease.

By defining those aspects of brain-mind states that are inaccessible to introspection as nonconscious, a huge area of psychology, philosophy, and psychoanalysis suddenly becomes amenable to unified scientific investigation. Today, a scientific psychology, a scientific philosophy, and a scientific psychoanalysis can all be solidly grounded in neurobiology.

This declaration will send shock waves through many institutionally embedded practitioners of psychology, philosophy, and psychoanalysis. They will see it as a threat, as a reduction of their field to neurobiology. Individual jobs are at stake, and in some cases university departments might be replaced. I would counsel against such panic on two counts. One is the conviction that each of these three fields will be *strengthened* by embracing the science of the nonconscious mind. Two is that the subsequent redefinition of each field is liberating, not enslaving, as many frightened practitioners would believe.

My vision of the redefinition of psychology, philosophy, and psychoanalysis has two aspects that should be quite attractive to those who do not want to go back to school to learn neurobiology. The first is that a great amount of work still needs to be done to develop a scientifically respectable phenomenology of the mind. We need more careful descriptions of mental processes via the properly limited use of introspection. We need catalogues of material describing normal and abnormal mental states that conform to the structure and goals of the mental status exam but which go beyond it both in detail and in time span. We need, for example, dream journals collected over a lifetime, and analysis of them; in all of my sixty years, I have not yet found one such journal. Psychology — that is, introspection — can be a powerful tool if it is used properly and within its own limits. But it must be recognized as part of a larger process, and not an end in itself.

The second attraction, and need, is to apply the proper tools of each field to a constructive critique of the new brain-mind paradigm. What does it mean to equate the nonconscious mind with the activation of brain cells? How must the brain sciences change to meet the opportunities and responsibilities of such a paradigm shift? What are the moral and ethical implications of recognizing that mental processes are material transactions between neurons? What are the proper humanistic frames of each viewpoint?

LEAVING SOME OF OUR LIVES TO CHANCE

Why should psychology, philosophy, and psychoanalysis want to make common cause with the brain sciences? Because all these fields have a shared interest in the same deep questions about human existence. To what extent are we part of a cosmic master plan? To what extent can our future be predicted by knowing our past? To what extent is the content of our thought at any moment derived from antecedent mental activity? And if we are going to give up the security of Biblical cosmology, Newtonian mechanics, and Freudian psychodynamics — all of which adhere to some form of strict determinism — what in the world are we to put in their place? The short answer is that our creativity and our freedom both depend upon randomness. And randomness appears to be an intrinsic aspect of brain function.

Indeed, one of the most distasteful ideas associated with modern science is that randomness is a major determinant of events in the cosmos, including the origin of life. To the horror of the theologians, it is asserted that life arose out of chaos by chance, without any supervisory direction. In the beginning, there was no Word, only cosmic noise. We all share a deep fear of believing that any part of our life, and especially our mental life, is subject to the whim of chance.

We prefer to think that all such processes obey strict, causal rules that are set by some architect who is as rational — but wiser — than ourselves. One reason for the surprising popularity of psychoanalysis is that it provides a sense of certainty and closure. Playing the game of life according to deterministic rules guarantees safety from the unexpected and the uncontrollable. Every dream is a wish whose fundamental impulse can be identified, understood, and controlled.

But what if the world has no beginning and no end? What if our minds are not directly knowable? How are we to live comfortably with such uncertainty? Who *is* in charge if not we or Him? Must we trust an *it*, a mechanism that is mental but not conscious? We balk at such an idea.

It is ironic that so many of us who profess to love freedom have so blindly embraced a psychology that offers the security of psychic determinism at the cost of the freedom that chance — and only chance — guarantees. The brain-mind paradigm offers us security via the reliability of our own cellular processes, yet guarantees us freedom through the unpredictability that these processes can bring. Yes, there is always the chance that we will die in our sleep because our breathing program will get stuck and just stop. Yes, there is always the chance that we will be walking down the street one day and just flip our lid. But the probability is extremely low.

Although these possibilities may be unnerving, they are good and quite necessary. Suppose all mental events were the predictable working of a machine so well engineered that it always functioned perfectly. How could creativity arise from such an automaton? How could novelty ever occur? It could not. Nature tinkers creatively via genetic mutation. Mutation, a chance event, is the most creative force in nature. Yet it is a horribly cruel force, since most mutations, like most of our ideas, are fatally flawed.

Nowhere is the role of chance more evident in our mental life than in dreams. By recognizing this truth, we acknowledge that dreaming occurs with predictable unpredictability. The nonconscious brain-mind is both highly reliable in its overall design and highly unpredictable in the details of its night-to-night operation.

Since each dream is created by the activation of 100 billion neurons in our brains, each connected to at least 10,000 others, and all chatter away at rates of up to 100 messages per second, how could we expect any other outcome than unpredictability of detail? A remarkable point is that some dreams do take up recurrent themes of undoubted significance to the life of the dreamer. Some seem to repeat almost exactly. How do we square this paradox? What part of dreaming is determined and what part is not?

The only answer we have is chaos. All complex systems — and the brain-mind is certainly a complex system — are characterized by a constant, dynamic interplay between chaos (unpredictability) and self-organization (orderliness). When we see orderliness, we tend to assume that it could be begotten only of orderliness — hence our naive acceptance of determinism.

Observe a stream of water or the flames above a fire and watch as orderly flow gives way to turbulence and then returns to orderliness again. In like fashion, our stream of consciousness flows, breaks, eddies, and reconvenes. In our innocence, we have tended to believe that all the breaks in the stream of our consciousness, whether during waking or dreaming, are meaningful. We must now admit that this is as unlikely an assumption as it is unproven. We must realize that dissociation is as much the rule of the brain-mind as association. And we should be thankful for it. Creativity separates us from most other animals, and it has its deep roots in the dissociative, chaotic nature of our nonconscious brain-minds.

ASSOCIATION AND DISSOCIATION

It is normal, even desirable, that our brain-mind states dissociate naturally. Within any state the processing of information is likely to be dissociated because the information is inherently jumpy, noisy, and discontinuous. The faculties that make up our states, such as memory or perception, may themselves be subject to the same kinds of inconsistencies and unpredictable changes. Without warning and without any identifiable stimulus, I may suddenly think of the name of a person I haven't seen or talked to in years. And I may imagine that person's face quite clearly.

We have already seen how our waking conscious can be dissociated into foreground and background processes. I can concentrate simultaneously on the mechanical act of shaving and the intellectual act of running through the day's upcoming events, in the foreground, while telling myself I look good in that mirror and playing out the dialogue that might unfold during any of my day's meetings, in the background. The foreground consists of perceptual data processing; the background consists of fantasy production. The fantasy itself ranges in content from literalness (the dialogue for the meetings) to abstractness (my self-image). The multiple and modular nature of the brain-mind contributes to all these levels of dissociation. Only the unity and constancy of the state-control system — the aminergic-cholinergic system — prevents this anarchic process from being more troublesome than it already is.

We know, too, that the brain-mind can be "split." The right hemisphere processes analogically and emotionally while the left hemisphere gives speech and narrative their logical form. The two hemispheres usually proceed harmoniously. But they can be dissociated from one another by cutting the corpus callosum, the large fiber bundle that connects the two hemispheres. When this is done, the subject's left brain cannot name the object that is seen by his right brain. The brain-mind can also be split so that the top is dissociated from the bottom. When a person sleepwalks, the cortext of his upper brain remains asleep while the lower brain is awake.

These dissociative experiences border on the maladaptive, and we therefore choose to call them disorders. But we should no longer regard dissociation as abnormal. Just as we should cheer chaos as essential to cognitive freedom and creativity, we should use our capacity to dissociate for health-supporting purposes. Hypnosis and meditation, for example, are effective because of dissociation; they enable a person to "tune out" the outside while remaining awake, thus reducing stress. These are voluntary changes of state that rely on dissociation to bring benefits.

Whenever we go to sleep we clearly abandon conscious control and let the nonconscious systems of our brain-mind do their automatic work. What the nonconscious brain-mind "decides" to do with each opportunity we cannot know. Here again, we need to abandon the idea that we can deduce a nonconscious cause for the information content of consciousness. They may be entirely dissociated phenomena.

At the same time that we recognize the shortcomings of the kind of psychological reductionism that was attempted by Freud, our scientific strategy of methodically studying the brain-mind one module at a time, or even one neuron at a time, is enormously enriched by realizing that in each investigation we have a good chance of learning something surprising, essential, and knowable in no other way. The brain-mind paradigm encourages an integration of psychology, psychoanalysis, and neurobiology. We should all be a bit more relaxed about demanding that the pieces fit together right away. In fact, at the rate we are progressing, we can expect to be in for a long haul. We have had access to what I am calling the nonconscious mind for only forty years. We have studied, at most, only a few thousand of those 100 billion neurons, an incredibly minuscule fraction. And very few of these were studied in a living human brain. We have a long way to go, but we are on the right track.

A CONSCIOUS DECISION
TO ALTER CONSCIOUSNESS

Nonetheless, there is just cause for celebration. We are finally beginning to get a glimpse of what is really going on inside our heads. We have only recently noticed that we are the embodiment of brain-mind states and that brain-mind states are all that we are. Our states control our faculties, yet with consciousness we can control our states.

Having cut consciousness down to size, let us end this discussion with enthusiasm for just how successfully it can still serve us. We can decide to pursue or not pursue the scientific study of our deep selves. We can decide to adopt or not adopt the brain-mind paradigm. I find the invitation, and my freedom to accept or refuse it, equally exciting.

If you decide to adopt the brain-mind paradigm, you have a powerful tool at your disposal, which you can use to improve your mental health. You can decide how best to condition your nonconscious and conscious brain-mind so that your vegetative life and your cognitive life can thrive and flourish. You can accomplish this by choosing which states your brain-mind may occupy and how long it may reside in any one state. Should you sleep more or less? Should you engage in meditation, hypnosis, or trance? In a parallel strategy, the mind doctors among us can decide how to manipulate the states of others, in order to help them. What is the best way to solve Bertal's problem and that of people who sleepwalk, or are depressed, or are addicts, and so on? These issues form the focus for Part Three.

CHANGING THE BRAIN-MIND

CHAPTER 13

How the Brain-Mind Heals
Itself

NOW THAT YOU HAVE a full understanding of how brain-mind state changes affect your faculties, and how subtle changes determine the differences between normal and abnormal states, it is time to use this powerful knowledge to your advantage. The final section of this book will show you how to begin.

This chapter explains how the brain-mind helps itself. The system has its own built-in healing power. If left to its own devices, the brain-mind is quite capable of correcting itself. Unfortunately, until you have a grasp of how it does so, you are as likely to interfere with the process as you are to help it.

The basic action that the brain-mind takes to keep itself fit is to change its state. You can improve your health — both mental and physical — by jostling the system a little, by voluntarily changing states to achieve certain effects. Techniques such as meditation, hypnosis, trance, and the placebo effect are among the acts of volition used by many "normal" people to change states and thus health. These are the subjects of chapter 14.

Of course some people are unable to exert such control. Others succumb to any one of a number of debilitating factors — psychological stress, addiction, chemical breakdown, disease, and the simple long-term death of cells. In these cases the system has to be jostled a lot. Drugs are often helpful in changing the brain-mind states of the "abnormal" people who fall into these situations. Only chemically induced changes in states can permanently heal them. However, as you will see in chapter 15, drugs alone are not the answer.

SCIENTIFIC HUMANISM

The power we all have to affect our own health is demonstrated by our collective response to one of our most familiar enemies: the common cold. Ask ten people how to beat a nagging cold and you'll probably get ten different answers: fruit juices, steam baths, chicken soup, vapor rubs — not to mention any one of an armful of over-the-counter nostrums available at the local pharmacy. But there is one remedy everyone agrees on: more sleep.

If you take sleep seriously enough, it helps more than any potion from the refrigerator or the drugstore. I have learned that for myself over the past two winters.

Three years ago a persistent cold turned nasty when I was in Sicily beginning to write this book. But since my time was my own, I was free to experiment with the sleep cure. Within a few days of going to bed at 10:00 P.M. and sleeping until 9:00 A.M. (instead of 12:00 till 7:00), my fatigue, lassitude, and evening cough were gone. Within a week I was completely well.

This past winter, by contrast, I was stateside and was struggling to squeeze my writing into an already busy schedule. As each hectic week evolved, I could feel my chest cold worsen. On the weekends, my Sicilian-style sleep-ins strengthened me enough so that on Monday I was close to being comfortable. Three extra hours of sleep were enough to knock the bug down, but not out. Finally the bug got the better of me, and off I went to three days of bed rest and sleep. Only then did I really begin to recover.

What's going on? Why is sleep the only cure that ultimately works? By sleeping so much, I am consciously shifting the balance of time my brain-mind and body spend in the energy-expensive ergotropic awake mode toward the more energy-conservative, and healing, trophotropic sleep mode. I am voluntarily manipulating my brain-mind states. And finally I get well.

The lesson here is that the brain-mind is good at healing itself, and that we can direct this healing by changing our brain-mind states. Furthermore, as we all know, the key to good health is not to get sick! The best way to increase the probability of staying well is to elect behaviors associated with health. The best doctor, then, is the self, the only agent who can engineer sound health practices.

This view, and its application to our mental and physical health, is something I call "scientific humanism." It recognizes a powerful top-down influence of cognition over the nonconscious states. Without appealing to forces outside the self, scientific humanism incorporates the power of positive thinking that is extolled by so many religions.

Scientific humanism is modest in its goals. It can't cure everything, and it is less grandiose in its cosmology. It has no God, no founding father (or mother), and no official healers. As a discipline, it places its highest reliance on the self as healer and views the states of the brain-mind as inherently health promoting. It says that the self (defined as an activated state of the brain-mind) extends to the whole body. To understand the self thoroughly requires an active interest in both traditional psychology and modern neurobiology.

Scientific humanism sees knowledge as more important than texts, ritual practice, or divinely inspired gurus, although it recognizes that much can be learned from the concepts and experiences of many charismatics, from William James to the Dalai Lama. It assumes that many important truths are already known but lie outside the usual realm of science, and that many more important truths remain to be established by the application of science to health practices.

Likewise, scientific humanism views the original goal of Sigmund Freud — to forge a scientific psychology — as entirely laudable. It sees neurobiology as a fundamental element in any reconstruction of psychoanalysis; it does not suppose that neurobiology would entirely replace or swallow up psychoanalysis. Scientific humanism also does not seek to disenfranchise physicians: a broken leg still requires a good orthopedic surgeon; pneumonia still requires an infectious disease specialist; and psychosis still requires the most sophisticated brain-mind psychiatrists. But scientific humanism *does* enfranchise, empower, and enjoin individuals to know more and to act more in the interest of their own health. It assumes, as many scientific epidemiologic studies have proven, that health is either the strong correlate or the direct causal consequence of practices that can be influenced and controlled by conscious decision making.

Of all the practices known to be associated with good health, sleep is the most fundamental. The most basic step you can take to improve your health is to figure out how much sleep you need and to see that you get it. As we have seen in every chapter of this book, the brain-mind seeks to regulate itself, and the best you can do is to let it do so. You have to discover your true sleep requirement, then help yourself to get it. Later in this chapter you will read about several cases that show that the brain-mind regulates itself by changing states, and that the most fundamental state change is from waking to sleeping. The cases show how some people need only a little sleep, some a lot and how we all run into trouble when we try to alter our natural tendency. They also show how, through simple evaluation and common sense practices, you can overcome sleep problems to improve your health.

There are three important reasons for focusing on sleep as the brain-mind's own resident physician. First, it is resident in that it is a built-in state change, and a physician in that its intrinsic healing mechanism has been detailed at the level of brain cells and molecules. The second is that its curative function is beginning to be specified as an enhancement to the immune system. And the third is that the mechanistic and functional rules that are emerging from sleep research can be extended to other curative conditions that are still on the fringe of science. Since the power of suggestion is notoriously strong, we can no longer afford to marginalize it as hysterical hocus-pocus. Instead, we must begin to harness its power.

FINDING YOUR SLEEP NICHE

"How much sleep do I need?" is a question I am asked all the time. Do you expect me to say 7.5 hours? I can't answer in that way. I can say that 7.5 hours is about average, but that is a purely statistical answer. It doesn't tell you if you are "average" or even if average folk are healthy. There is no quick answer. Only a month or so of careful self-observation can tell you convincingly whether or not you are getting enough sleep. Bear in mind, too, that the amount you need can change with age, lifestyle, and illness.

The clinical approach to sleep evaluation — and one I've adopted personally — begins with a simple chart. I'll describe how the method tracks both the quantity and quality of sleep, and you can adapt it for yourself.

What's needed is a grid on a wide piece of paper. I number days from 1 to 30 down the left-hand edge of the paper. Each day gets its own row running across the page from left to right. Across the top of the page I list each hour of the day, from 12:00 noon one day (at the left) to 12:00 noon the next day (at the right). Each hour gets its own column running down the page from the top to bottom. With a light pencil mark I divide each hour into quarters.

Each day I mark the time I went to bed (to the nearest quarter hour), the time I actually fell asleep, the times during the night I got up, and the time I woke up in the morning. Using a felt-tip pen I draw a line connecting the time I fell asleep with the time I woke up. As the days progress down the page, a bar chart emerges indicating the number of hours I sleep.

During the waking hours of each day, I use a series of codes to note any unpleasant changes in my level of attention (A) or in my energy flow (F), and to note the time of occurrence of meals (M), exercise (E), sexual activity (S), alcohol intake (I), and tobacco use (T). In parallel with this rather dull and quantitative procedure I keep a narrative journal in which I record my dreams (because they interest and amuse me), as well as qualitative notes about how I felt each day, whom I spent time with, and whatever philosophical or quasi-artistic inspirations I might have had.

Taken together, my sleep chart and journal give me a detailed picture of my nonconscious and conscious states. Sometimes it is difficult to say whether I slept well because I felt good or whether I felt good because I slept well. But it really doesn't matter. What is clear is that when I don't sleep well I don't feel good. What is most useful about documenting the details is that I can look back to see what my behavior was before my bad nights and what kind of nights preceded bad days.

In order to feel healthy, I need a total of seven to nine hours of sleep a night; a prompt sleep onset of no more than thirty and usually less than ten minutes; no more than three awakenings of no more than five minutes each; a regular time of going to bed (between 10:30 and 11:30 P.M.); and a regular time of rising (between 6:30 and 7:00 A.M.). You may need more or less. You have only to be honest with yourself and exert some modest discipline to find out.

In addition, several factors conspire to confound my sleep. Alcohol intake and overeating, especially when they occur together, delay the onset of my sleep, cause me to sleep fitfully, and result in poor alertness the next morning. A failure to exercise, which in my case is often related to an overabsorption in work, has the same effect.

From this straightforward set of observations it is obvious what I need to do to get and stay on the health track: eat breakfast, be sure to take a daily swim or run, avoid more than a glass of wine or two, and get the full seven to nine hours of sleep.

This exercise in self-observation and the changes I make as a result together constitute a simple example of how an individual can improve and control his health using the brain-mind paradigm. By committing myself to the self-observation practice, I focus my attention on the aspects of my behavior that improve my sleep state and therefore improve one of my faculties — my attention — during my waking state. By engaging in this process, I am engaging my conscious mind to be causal on my health, via its effects on my nonconscious mind (the sleep state). Here we see that this grand paradigm and all its seeming complexities can be quite obvious and simple to use.

IT'S NORMAL TO BE ABNORMAL

The sleep prescription I have given myself works only for me. You will have to do your own analysis to find a prescription for yourself. As you plot the outcome, don't be surprised by extremes. There is great variation in our nonconscious states; some people need very little sleep, others need a great deal, and many people require more (even if just a little bit more) than the social world allows. Which means we must either change the social world, invest more heartily in genetic engineering, or change our own conscious approach to controlling our states. Obviously, only the last option is realistic, so let's take it.

The uniqueness of each individual's states was made clear to me recently, as I was beginning to yawn at the end of an elaborate and endless dinner meeting. My colleague Lia Sylvestri, who usually has more spunk than I do at such a late juncture in the day, seemed to lack her usual brilliance on this particular occasion. I already knew Lia was a short sleeper; she was often able to function impressively with as few as one and a half to three hours of sleep.

"How much sleep did you get last night?" I asked her.

"Thirty minutes," she said.

When I asked her if she was tired now, she admitted that she was. "How much sleep will you get tonight?" I asked.

"Three to five hours," she replied, making me feel a bit more like I was talking to someone from my own planet and not a bionic superwoman designed by a genetic engineer.

Lia is a typical short sleeper. She is active and productive in her career as a neurologist specializing in sleep and movement disorders, and as a woman who is raising two young children with her present spouse and four older ones from a previous marriage. She is competent, happy, and well liked in both roles. She exhibits no evidence of being pathologically anxious or hypomanic, as one might expect of even short sleepers with such a demanding life.

"Could you sleep longer if you tried?" I asked.

"Oh sure," she asserted. "Whenever I like."

And indeed, the scientific evidence is with her on that point.

Young students who volunteer for my sleep lab can sleep longer, by choice, if I offer to pay $5 an hour for each hour of bona fide sleep they exhibit. Some students, so motivated, can double their sleep time. That's certainly good news for insomniacs — they just need to find someone to pay them for sleeping. (Actually, insomniacs can set up a Skinnerian reward system for themselves; it sometimes works!)

But Lia really threw me for a loop when she added, "Before I had children, I slept as much as anyone else."

Lia's idea that her current pattern was simply a product of habit seemed highly unlikely to me — and I still don't believe it. I think she is, and always was, a genetically determined short sleeper who *increased* her sleep length when she was an adolescent, to fit in with societal and family norms. Lia's spouse, Raoul di Perri, who is every bit as friendly and hardworking as his wife, agrees. He lives in the same household, with the same six children, but sleeps eight to nine hours a night. All attempts to drastically shorten his sleep have failed dismally.

Most short sleepers say that they always knew they needed less sleep than their peers. When Lia gets three to four hours of sleep, she is fine and can go at it full tilt for the twenty or twenty-one hours she is awake. When she gets less, she does tire. Although she can sleep longer, she usually doesn't; Lia has a genuine capacity to significantly curtail her sleep without any negative effect. On a rare weekend she may indeed choose to sleep longer (relatively speaking). She's not "catching up" on her sleep when she does so, however; she just wants a bit of peace and quiet away from her otherwise busy work and home life.

Lia is the only child of a couple with sleep propensities that suggest a strong genetic determination of her own short sleep. Her mother has always been a light, fitful sleeper and now, at age seventy-five, still sleeps only five to six hours a night. This is not terribly striking. But her father, Enzo, is another story. A professor of real estate law, Enzo is still vigorous and productive at age seventy-eight, and feels rested after only three to four hours of sleep. Most significant is his capacity to turn sleep on and off like a faucet. If he feels a bit tired, he can promptly fall asleep — anywhere — and then awaken twenty minutes later fully restored and ready for action.

As a culture that strongly values activity and accomplishment, we naturally envy genetically short sleepers, who typically can accomplish more in a day than those of us who need more sleep. This cultural bias leads us to make several important mistakes that need to be more clearly recognized and dealt with both by individuals who need a lot of sleep and by society at large, which tends to devalue sleep.

Several times I have put ads in the Boston papers looking for people who sleep less than five or more than nine hours every day, and each time I received numerous responses. For every Lia and Enzo in the world there is a person who needs more sleep than the 7.5-hour average. But his or her chances of getting it, or being understood, are slim. One such person was Rosa, a medical student of mine, who admitted at age twenty-seven that she felt completely rested only after fourteen hours of sleep. You can imagine how much she enjoyed her internship.

In all likelihood Rosa did not actually need fourteen hours of sleep every night. But she might well have needed nine to eleven hours, and complained that she needed fourteen because she was chronically sleep deprived by always limiting her sleep to make it match the seven- to eight-hour societal norm and her own tough medical schedule. Families, spouses, friends, and employees just do not accept the reality of a long sleeper's needs. The long sleepers of the world are every bit as much social pariahs as the Lias and Enzos are heroes.

Lazy, sleepy-head, and good-for-nothing are a few of the unflattering epithets that are heaped on those unfortunates. This reinforcement is really a kind of punishment. Long sleepers would often prefer to be called narcoleptics or even depressives to help them legitimize their legitimate need. Long sleepers are as natural as tall people. Unfortunately, our society has not created a sport as respected or well paid as basketball for those who sleep tall.

The social stigma attached to long sleepers in work-ethic cultures is not softened by the fact that long sleepers are not particularly energetic even during their abbreviated waking hours. Many of them may be lethargic and introverted, whereas Lia and Enzo are energetic and outgoing. To their close friends, however, the long sleepers may be quite appealing because they tend to be more sensitive, poetic, and receptive than the go-getter short sleeper types.

Where do you stand on this spectrum, which stretches from two to fourteen hours and clusters at about 7.5? Unless you make a conscious effort, you'll never get a chance to find out. As William Wordsworth pointed out, "The world is too much with us; late and soon/Getting and spending we lay waste our powers:/Little we see in Nature that is ours." As an intrinsic part of scientific humanism, we should consider better treatment of our own bodies and develop a more natural approach to our nonconscious brain-minds. Attaining good health is your own responsibility, and you can control it to a great degree by consciously investigating and manipulating your brain-mind states.

THE THOMAS EDISON SYNDROME

What happens if you don't take control? You inevitably end up fighting the system. As a result, you might simply feel tired all the time. But much more debilitating and obsessive fates can befall you.

This conclusion not only applies to sleep, it applies to a vast range of human behaviors, dependent on brain-mind states, that must move uneasily between biological reality and egalitarian delusion. Long and short sleepers are born, not made, but they have to fit their genetic predisposition into one societal niche or another. If you are miscast, you have to find a way to reduce the gaps between native constitution and social expectation. Otherwise, you might end up like Edwin.

Edwin is the founder, owner, and president of a small electronics company that operates out of his garage in the suburbs of Turner's Falls, Massachusetts, once a prosperous mill town that is fast falling into poverty. Despite possessing twenty-six patents on printed circuit boards and the related entrails of servo-gadgets that might one day allow him to rocket his kitchen to the moon, Edwin's business is foundering.

He is convinced that a major reason for his failure as an entrepreneur is his excessive need for sleep, and not long ago he consulted me for treatment of what he himself had confidently diagnosed as a typical case of narcolepsy. Not surprisingly, Edwin reads the *Wall Street Journal* and had encountered several detailed descriptions therein of sleep disorders. According to some alarmist advocates of sleep disorder medicine, almost half the citizens of the United States are suffering from one or more of the three hundred syndromes that have been recently described by sleep laboratory scientists.

Edwin does have excessive daytime sleepiness, the most common and annoying symptom that narcoleptics complain of, and he is sometimes extremely sleepy at meetings with prospective financial backers and technical collaborators. Meticulous, well-dressed, even dapper, Edwin described his symptoms in minute detail as if I were a patent examiner instead of a physician, and as if he wanted to convince me both of the validity and originality of his claim.

In fact, Edwin believed that with the proper medication he would be able to turn his company around and take advantage of the economic boom that was "just around the corner." Furthermore, he had decided that the proper medication was Ritalin, an amphetamine-like drug that mimics the action of norepinephrine (which we know boosts our alertness and energy flow). Edwin had read that the antidepressants might also be effective in treating narcolepsy, but, because he clearly was not depressed, he said he would prefer a stimulant medication. I agreed that such a drug would probably give Edwin quite a lift, but at what cost? I was also not so sure he was not depressed. Given his story it would certainly be understandable.

I asked if he ever felt so irresistibly sleepy that he literally dropped in his tracks? No, not really, he said. He could usually fight off his somnolence so that no one noticed it, and he had never suddenly lost control of his muscles as occurs in the so-called cataleptic attacks of narcolepsy. Since these collapses of postural tone are often triggered by surprise, laughter, or strong positive emotions, such as joy or erotic excitement, I asked if his sleepiness was ever prompted by emotion. No, he said, and added that he rarely experienced emotion. He was too rational and too busy for that sort of foolishness.

You can imagine how little weight he placed on such a whimsical phenomenon as dreaming.

"Can't remember any dreams ever!" he said, when I began a line of inquiry about bad dreams at sleep onset, which are part of the narcolepsy picture. Nor did he ever wake up from a dream unable to move, so he had no sleep paralysis. Quite the contrary, he often awakened quickly and leaped out of bed to jot down a possible patentable invention idea. I asked Edwin whether he thought his brain-mind ever really had any time off. He smiled, as if I were on to something, and said, "You know, I really feel that sleep is a waste of time and that I shouldn't need it at all."

"Wherever did you get that idea?" I asked. Edwin was the latest of five similar cases of self-diagnosed narcolepsy that I had seen. I suddenly began to wonder whether he might have absorbed his views about his physical condition from the media, like many of my female medical students, who have been taught by the media that attractiveness is achieved only by being thin and so have starved and even purged themselves in a vain attempt to look like Twiggy. Could it be that Edwin was on a self-imposed diet of sleep starvation? Suppose he was a completely normal sleeper who was trying to force himself to be a short sleeper?

To my utter amazement, Edwin then treated me to a detailed description of the sleep habits of his hero, Thomas Edison, inventor-entrepreneur par excellence. Edison's modest needs for sleep and his ability to sleep anywhere, anytime (for example, under the stairs of his Menlo Park laboratory) are legendary, even if they have never been documented. Then it suddenly occurred to me that whether the story is legend or myth hardly matters now that Edison is gone. His image lives on and inspires the Edwins of the world to emulate Edison's talents, including his brief and efficient sleep.

When I suggested this idea to Edwin, he readily confirmed his own conscious adoption of Edison as his role model. At our next session he brought me a huge file on Edison, along with his own carefully documented sleep log. There was Edison, the inventor of the lightbulb, a man who hardly needed to sleep; here was Edwin, limiting his sleep to as little as four hours per night, then feeling tired all day. The condensation of ideas made my head swim. I realized that Edwin was not the only one suffering from the Edison syndrome, as I came to call this series of cases: all of us were.

We all feel inadequate (to varying degrees) if we are not creative, entrepreneurial, wealthy, and continuously wakeful. Many of us may wish we could eliminate the need for sleep entirely. Indeed, why not give Edwin the chemical boost his relatively normal brain needed to realize the short sleep program he had imposed on it? It certainly would have been an easier course than the one I embarked on, which was to try to change Edwin's behavior in a more natural-istic way by changing both his mind and his sleep habits.

Part of my reason for choosing this route came from the bad experiences I had encountered in the psychoactive medication craze I was immersed in during its heyday in the 1960s. And part of it came from my revulsion toward the extensive reliance on tech-nology that seemed to me to be alienating the medical profession from the most personal aspect of its obligation to patients — to deeply care about the quality of their lives.

We do not need drugs to sleep well. In small farm towns, no one is motivated to curtail their sleep. The simplemindedness of the farm community is right on target. If someone needs to sleep more, they should go to bed earlier and sleep more. Period. Fur-thermore, farm folks are able to sleep better because both their minds and bodies exist in a more natural environment. City life has driven us away from the natural sleep enhancers — physical work, clean air, and low stress. The modern ethic — that sleep is a waste of time and should be eliminated by science — is clearly a by-product of industrialization and of the elaboration of behav-ioral norms that serve it; not that a long sleeper would be a popular member of a farm family. There is much hard work to be done.

But the family would tolerate the deviance, because natural aberration and even disaster are more easily accommodated by agrarian societies.

Another important contribution to my own naturalistic philosophy of brain-mind state management came from my service years ago on a National Science Foundation commission formed by the Food and Drug Administration to evaluate the efficacy of electrosleep machines. Soviet scientists had the idea that sleep could be induced and enhanced through electric currents and had designed a device to carry out the task.

If Edwin had gotten his hands on one of these gizmos, he might have patented it and retired rich. The idea would have appealed to him. The notion was to create a supersleep by electrically stimulating the brain with a device worn on the head. It was assumed that sleep efficiency, or depth, or whatever could be doubled.

Clearly, both the capitalist and communist philosophies are infected with the same virus: that we should not need to sleep; or, at the very least, that we should need to sleep less. For the Soviets, this engineering was natural to central planners. Their willingness to abuse science in the interest of Lenin-like schemes for progress was well known. One obvious reason for the failure of the Soviet five-year plans for factory production was the eight-hour workday. Why not increase the endurance of the workers to twelve hours by buzzing his brain and thereby reducing his sleep by the four hours needed to make up the difference?

Fortunately for all of us, the electrosleep machine didn't work. Not only did it fail to produce supersleep, it didn't even enhance normal sleep. We canned the idea as unfeasible and the contraption as unreliable. The American people had been spared at least one bit of pseudoscientific gimmicky. If only we could be as effective in rooting out the antisleep software of our society! By that I mean the hyperwork ethic, the type A personality syndrome, the way of daily life that keeps so many people so turned on they can't turn off even when they try. Powerfully vested cultural and commercial interests conspire to promote the infection of your brain-mind just as they did that of Edwin.

I didn't have much luck in my effort to convince Edwin that

no amount of modern biochemical ingenuity could turn him into Thomas Edison. I tried to get him to realize that he was no Edison, at least when it came to sleep requirements. I tried to persuade him to use his sleep chart as a guide to increasing the time spent asleep. He heard, but he didn't listen. He had attached himself to an ideal of achievement and he wouldn't return to the solid ground of reality. And since I was unwilling to turn Edwin into an amphetamine addict, he left in disgust. I suspect, I am sorry to say, that he had no difficulty convincing another physician that he really did have narcolepsy and that he really did need drugs.

PHYSICIAN, HEAL THYSELF!

My resistance to prescribing drugs for Edwin sprang in part from my experience with Dr. George Lowell, a medical colleague of mine in the 1970s who had diagnosed himself as narcoleptic years earlier when he was in medical school, because he was often sleepy during lectures. If falling asleep in medical school lectures was an adequate criterion for the diagnosis of narcolepsy, all doctors would be patients. There was no more convincing evidence that Dr. Lowell was narcoleptic than there was in Edwin's case. He was a long, or even normal, sleeper who had been cast by his choice of a medical career in a short-sleeper's role. But he prescribed himself stimulants *and* antidepressants and took them for years. He became addicted. Over time he became unmanageable. His hospital position was put in jeopardy, and his marriage became rocky.

Watching Dr. Lowell disintegrate helped convince me that I needed to develop an even more affirmative education program for my colleagues than the one I had designed for my patients. I needed to better educate my young students about the brain-mind paradigm and the virtues of a naturalistic approach. I also needed to warn my colleagues and students against mistaking natural and normal responses to stress for diseases (or even disorders) and, whatever the problem, against self-diagnosis, self-treatment, and self-prescription.

Since that time, I have always accepted invitations to lecture to young medical students to try to break this vicious cycle at its inception. After one such session, in North Carolina, a young student who has since become a colleague asked me if I would see his father, a physician, who had suffered for years from intractable insomnia. With modest admonishments against false hopes, I said yes. The case was special, but it illustrates how genetics, life events, culture, and personality all conspire to make a natural course of sleep improbable.

The story illustrates how education, behavior modification, persistence, and goodwill can successfully counter these powerful negative forces. It also illustrates how, through simple evaluation and change, an individual can alter his brain-mind states to improve his health.

It was easy to persuade Dr. Larry Richberg that his excessive daytime sleepiness was not due to narcolepsy. He knew that he was sleep deprived, owing to insomnia, and he knew that his insomnia was caused by anxiety. One thing that struck Dr. Richberg as odd was that although he had always been a relatively light sleeper (a genetic predisposition), he could always sleep better on Friday and Saturday nights than on weeknights (an environmental factor). He had also noticed that Sunday was the worst night of the week, especially if he was to play an active role the next day at his hospital's weekly medical board meeting (a specific psychological factor).

Dr. Richberg's sleep charts were as meticulous as Edwin's, but his self-observation journal was helpful, too. Dr. Richberg had taken care to note the psychologically idiosyncratic workings of his own mind. The particular factor affecting his sleep pattern was his fear of defeat, failure, and rejection in his professional work. Earlier in his career he had lost his position at a major hospital center. This blow to his self-esteem was countered by his subsequent success in a private hospital nearby, but his sense of autonomy and security was constantly undermined by an uneasy competitiveness with Dr. Frank Cutter, a surgical colleague bent upon taking Dr. Richberg's space, his equipment, his trainees, and his billings. Sad to say, this is not an uncommon scenario.

I saw Dr. Richberg a total of twenty times over a three-year period during which he made major gains in the management of his anxiety, his maladaptive behavior at work, and his sleep. The key steps that he took involved all the well-documented natural aids to sleep, as well as some specially tailored moves that fit his particular situation. Together, he and I came up with the following prescription.

Sleep When Tired

One of the boldest moves Dr. Richberg made was to install a couch in his office at the hospital. He is not a psychoanalyst. But he could close the door each day after lunch and take a nap if needed. In this way he gained relief from and control of his sleepiness.

Get Up When Wakeful

Dr. Richberg loved classical music, so instead of lying hopelessly awake in bed in the grips of tense, rumination anxiety, he went to his den and listened to a symphony. This relaxed him enough to go back to sleep within twenty to thirty minutes.

Practice the Relaxation Response

Both at work and in bed, Dr. Richberg learned to listen to his breathing, to count his slow deep breaths, and to allow the muscle tension to flow from his limbs. In doing so, he interrupted the flow of energy from his brain to his body, which reduced the flow of energy from his body to his brain.

Exercise

Before consulting me Dr. Richberg had suffered a serious heart attack, which understandably had made him quite frightened of overtaxing his healing heart. His cardiologist and I agreed, however, that both his heart and his sleep would benefit from moderate exercise: a two-mile walk in the late afternoon or early evening.

Tobacco and Alcohol

Never a smoker and not much of a drinker, Dr. Richberg learned to enjoy a glass of sherry with his wife before dinner as another way of being sure to separate his work life from his recreation and his rest.

Sex

This particularly pleasurable form of exercise brought Dr. Richberg and his wife both intimacy and a natural sleep readiness. Prostate surgery had caused his ejaculations to flow backward into his bladder, a convenient and amusing contraceptive technique that he learned to laugh about. His cardiologist and I both endorsed his resumption of this instinctive and exciting behavior.

Breakfast

Taking time in the morning to begin his day at breakfast with his wife was an important way of ending his night of sleep on a pleasant and positive note. Instead of rushing off to the hospital unreadied, malnourished, and tense, he began his day calm, well-fed, and refreshed.

Stop Telling Ethnic Jokes

Dr. Richberg, who is Jewish, had the habit of regaling Dr. Cutter, an Irish Catholic, with jokes about Jesus, the Pope, and Richard Nixon. Dr. Cutter was not amused. By telling these jokes in poor taste, Dr. Richberg was validating his own sense of himself as a compulsive clown, born to lose, which was the major subject of his insomniac fantasies. He posted an invisible sign on the inside of his forehead that read: "No jokes!"

There is nothing a physician wants more than an appropriately grateful patient, someone who gets well with a little help, but mostly on his own. While it might not have done harm to add temporary use of sleep medication to the natural regimen, it was unnecessary, and both Dr. Richberg and I were interested to see how far we could go without it. I think we both wanted his son to see that, too.

Today, Dr. Richberg sleeps like a baby — most of the time. He is radiantly happy with the results. He is clear and calm and his medical practice is doing quite well. And his sleep problem was significant. If he could cure himself, those of us who have occasional bouts with lesser sleep problems can surely do the same.

The point is: Yes, a solution can be that simple. Dr. Richberg had tried every conventional cure — medication, psychoanalysis, and more — and nothing had worked. When he simplified his life, he got better. There was no gimmick, no machine, no deep secret.

This is a curious statement for me to make, but: Many times people think too much. They think that problems must require complex solutions. Many times, a return to fundamentals is all that's needed. Dr. Richberg is now fine. Dr. Lowell is taking every pill in sight and is losing his marriage, his career, and his life. I shudder to think how frazzled Edwin must be by now. Rosa, the long-sleeping medical student, is still persecuted by society, and she's still tired. My colleague Lia, the short sleeper, is sharp as ever. I found a sleep cure for my colds and have used it successfully ever since, without wasting my money at the drugstore.

One way to sum up the message of all these bedtime stories is to say that the brain knows best. It knows what it needs, it knows how to get it, and it knows what to do once its needs are met. Sleep is of the brain, by the brain, for the brain. And it benefits the body as well. But the naturally beneficial effects of sleep can occur only if we let them occur. Sometimes our managerial selves won't allow them to happen. In that event, we may need to consult another manager to learn the special state-control techniques like hypnosis that are detailed in the next chapter. If that fails, we may finally need to resort to the chemical manipulation of the brain-mind state-control system that we will look into in the last chapter.

CHAPTER 14

Changing Brain-Mind States to Improve Your Health

ISSOCIATIVE brain-mind states that rely on the power of suggestion are often dismissed as a sham. Hypnosis is ridiculed as a hoax, trance as a fake, meditation as nothing more than relaxation, multiple personality as playacting. Even lucid dreaming is in danger of being scuttled on the shoals of scientific respectability. Here's the paradox, though: almost every doctor and scientist would agree that the placebo effect works on some people. Well, what is the placebo effect? The power of suggestion.

Taken in its broadest form, the power of suggestion is indeed a powerful tool that we all can use to alter our brain-mind states and improve our health. When we suggest to ourselves, we are acting out of free will. The voluntary changing of state is an act of volition, an act of self-suggestion. Meditation, trance, and hypnosis can be induced by all of us if we believe it is possible. We can use these three altered states to change our health.

DENTAL SURGERY UNDER HYPNOSIS

Lest you doubt it, consider the success of Dr. Robert Drury. I met Bob in 1961, after my disillusionment with psychoanalysis and my horror over the Korean War prompted me to move from my residency with Harvard Medical School at The Psycho to the National Institutes of Health, in Bethesda, Maryland. There I was able to pursue a scientific education while fulfilling my military obligation as a member of the U.S. Public Health Service Commissioned Corps. During my first year my responsibilities were mainly clinical: I took medical care of a group of schizophrenic patients who were the subjects of an intensive research project on biochemical causes of mental disorders. I also provided psychiatric consultation to patients in the National Cancer Institute, many of whom were dying and in extreme physiological and psychological pain.

Bob was a young dentist, and his practice turned out to be extremely influential in my thinking. His job was to provide dental care for the research subjects in my schizophrenia unit. I was impressed with how easily he was able to obtain cooperation for invasive dental procedures from these very confused, sometimes flagrantly paranoid, and often stubbornly resistant patients. When I asked him how he did it, he told me he was a trained hypnotist.

I was as skeptical as the average physician. I asked Bob plainly if he thought hypnosis was real. "Come to the dental clinic and I'll show you," he suggested.

Before the visit could be arranged, we got together for supper and, at my suggestion, Bob put several of the guests into a light trance. He induced their arms to float up weightlessly and prompted them to enact some innocent posthypnotic suggestions, like getting up and turning off the lights. I had seen this sort of "stage" hypnosis before, and I have seen it many times since. The histrionic quality of these performances only made me more skeptical. It is this clear collusion between hypnotist and subject that has prompted criticism of the validity of hypnosis as an authentic mental state. And, indeed, the charge of fakery is difficult to dismiss in these scenarios.

In the dental clinic, however, there was a more scientifically cogent reason for believing that the hypnosis Dr. Drury induced was real. He used hypnosis instead of anesthesia to help patients block pain. The patients could have been faking, but if they were, their fakery was effective — on themselves. If they could fool themselves into thinking they didn't feel pain, then what kind of pain did they have? Hypnotic anesthesia worked, and it worked by dissociation.

On the day I attended the clinic, Dr. Drury was performing a painful gum excision on a patient with gingivitis. Anyone who has undergone a gingivectomy will tell you it is not a pleasant procedure. The patient was not a schizophrenic, and he was not the usual stage-trance type either. He was a healthy no-nonsense sailor who worked as a medical technician across Wisconsin Avenue at the Bethesda Naval Hospital. With Bob's encouragement, he had learned to prefer hypnosis to Novocain as a way of achieving dental anesthesia.

Bob's demonstration of hypnosis was dramatic. He first put the sailor into a moderately deep trance. He then suggested that the right side of the sailor's mouth, but not the left, would be insensitive to pain. When Bob probed the left gum with his needle-sharp pick, the sailor jumped and howled. But when he jabbed the gum on the right side, the sailor gave no response, even though the pick drew blood. Bob proceeded to cut away the compromised tissue with his scalpel. Hypnosis, I noted, had no effect on hemorrhage: there was plenty of bleeding. Yet the sailor sat there quietly.

Was this patient faking? Did the sailor really feel the pain but say he didn't? Did one part of the sailor feel the pain (his nonconscious brain-mind) while another part didn't (the conscious brain-mind)? Or was he able to turn off even his nonconscious brain-mind so that the stimuli were not even processed as pain? We don't yet know the answers to these important questions. But I can tell you this: the sailor was calm, relaxed, and wide awake throughout a painful procedure. Somewhere along the path from stimulus to response, the neuron signals were blocked. It didn't occur in the tissue: the gum was bleeding, so a pain signal was headed for the brain. Either the signal wasn't processed, or the motor response to it was blocked. We need more research to find out. Perhaps hypnosis blocks pain processing in the thalamus, a relay station for messages from the body to the brain. If this were the case, the hypnosis action would resemble that of lucid dreaming, in which a top-down signal (from the cortex) overrides a bottom-up signal (from the brain stem).

If you lend any credence to the brain-mind paradigm (and I imagine that if you don't you will not have reached this point in the book), the idea that we can voluntarily alter our physiological responsiveness to pain should not seem that outlandish. We know full well that when we daydream, internally generated visions replace externally generated ones. With this simple act we are controlling perception. Why, then, should we not be able to redirect attention from external to internal so that pain stimuli are either cancelled or denied access to the higher levels of our consciousness? Sure, it might be a more difficult task — ignoring an external pain signal requires more volition than ignoring external light waves — but the process is exactly the same. We are shifting states to alter a faculty. We are shifting the input source in the AIM model from external to internal. And that is all. Just because it might be harder to do doesn't mean it can't be done. Those of us with common sense are amazed at the resistance put up by psychologists, physiologists, and philosophers to the obvious reality of free will and the voluntary control of our bodies.

ITCH, BE GONE!

A critic might say that the sailor didn't feel pain in his gum because it was diseased. I later entertained this as a possible objection, as well as others, but the profuse bleeding couldn't be ignored. I did wonder, however, how far the approach could be taken. Could even outspoken disbelievers in hypnosis be induced to ignore physical discomfort? I soon learned they could.

The doctors of the National Cancer Institute were at their wits' end for many reasons, all related to the devastating consequences of cancer on their patients. One symptom that was particularly resistant to control was itching of the skin caused by the invasion of Hodgkin's lymphoma cells. I was asked to work with the patients who had this problem; some were driven almost to insanity by the itching, threatening to jump out of the windows of the cancer institute, which was on the eleventh floor.

I quickly realized that what these patients needed was a dentist named Drury, not a psychiatrist named Hobson, because the den-

tist was trained in hypnosis and the psychiatrist was a hypno-
phobe. I asked the patients, one by one, if they thought hypnosis
was "real." All ten said flatly that it was not. One tough old codger
from the Deep South, who had a glare in his eye and a piney drawl
to match the best of them, was literally tearing his cancer-riddled
skin apart trying to stop the itching. He was covered with antibiot-
ics to prevent infection of his broken skin. "Look here, boy," he
twanged at me, "you better put me to sleep before I do it myself!"

That gave me an idea. What about plain old sleep? The nurses
said that some of the patients did stop scratching at night (implying
abatement of the itch) but that others woke up more excoriated
than before they went to sleep (indicating that sleep scratching is a
real threat). The fact that we all are naturally anesthetic when we
sleep, and that we almost never experience pain in our dreams,
indicates clearly that a natural change in brain-mind state could
change the perception of an unpleasant stimulus (the itching) or
eliminate a damaging response to it (the scratching).

So I asked the patients, "If there was any chance that hypnosis
would help you, would you give it a try?"

"I'm sure I can't be hypnotized, but I'll try anything" was the
typical reply.

Enter Bob Drury. He came at my request, and one by one he
hypnotized the ten patients and told them they wouldn't itch and
shouldn't scratch. I didn't witness all ten attempted hypnotisms,
but I can tell you the outcome. Five of the patients had very significant relief. They were free of itching and scratching for three
weeks, after a single hypnotic session of about twenty minutes'
duration. One of those five was the tough old codger, and he was
as surprised as I.

What happened? Were these people faking? Hardly. They
wanted relief badly, badly enough to believe the hypnosis could
help.

Pain and itching are both subjective experiences. And hypnosis
relies on the power of suggestion. Like being "under the influence"
of alcohol, people can be "under the influence" of suggestion. And
as they do with alcohol, they change state very significantly under
the influence of suggestion. If we could just find the chemical or

electrical neural mechanisms that are triggered when people are under the influence of suggestion, we could put this powerful and useful technique on solid scientific ground. As one consequence, hypnosis could be integrated with mainstream medicine. We could then help many patients who are hypnotizable but don't know it because it has never been tried on them. As another consequence, we might be able to induce the hypnotic state physiologically, and so help even those patients who are not susceptible to suggestion.

THE BRAIN-MIND IN TRANCE

Throughout history, and in many parts of the world today, a brain-mind state called trance plays a central role in religious rituals. Among tribal people in Malaysia, for example, the trance state is called Latah.

Because trance can be induced by hypnosis, I will look closely at Latah, and some other exotic behaviors that share properties with it, in search of common underlying mechanisms that will help us begin to link them to our model of brain-mind state control. I will show how genetics, brain disorder, and culture can all conspire to predispose people to undergo rapid and dramatic changes in state. The fact that so many cultures use trance as an integral part of healing practices gives this comparative survey its relevance to our quest for ways in which health can be improved by altering states.

Like Drury's dental trance, Latah seems to have an anesthetic effect. When subjects have put themselves in a suitable trance state, their noses, ears, and cheeks are pierced with sharp skewers, which may then remain in place for a lifetime, as totemic inspiration to others in search of more intimate contact with the spirit world.

Not everyone is capable of the deep trance necessary to bear the ritual or the heavy weight of ornaments that are later added to the skewers. But everyone indulges in long hours of ritual practice. Ritual preparation, including intense dancing and sleep deprivation, begins many days before the public exhibition.

Some Malaysians are particularly susceptible to trance. If they are startled or tickled, they undergo a dramatic state change that is as rapid and distinctive as the cataleptic attacks of narcolepsy. But instead of their bodies falling limp and their minds falling into the dream state, as they would in REM sleep, they become hypnotically dissociated. It's as if someone flipped a switch and they suddenly lost contact with reality. They may utter unseemly streams of invectives or become submissively obedient to commands. The Latah trance is a hypersuggestible state that is itself suggested. But unlike hypnosis, it is triggered by a startle stimulus.

There is thus a potentially informative similarity between the use of Latah to bear the pain of the piercing ritual and the analgesia of hypnosis. Both require preparation by an agent (the priest or hypnotist). Both are states for which certain individuals have a heightened susceptibility. And both are experienced as a temporary abandonment of voluntary control in the interest of attaining a state through which personal or social well-being is enhanced. It appears there are two routes to the altered brain-mind state of trance. One is top-down, for which a hypnotist or shaman and some ritual is necessary. The other is bottom-up, requiring only a simple but sudden physical stimulus.

By either route the subject's brain-mind is seized and his perceptions and motor behavior are dramatically altered. The subject's private experience, especially pain perception, is changed drastically. The subject's control of both internal and external attention is lost. These perceptual and attentional features are similar to our own normal experience in fantasy and dreaming. They're just more dramatic.

We have already noted that when the hypnotist or priest induces trance, the subject's volition is surrendered in the interest of a personal or social goal. Because the processing of external data and the orienting response depend on the posterior (rear) region of the cortex, we might suppose that during hypnotic induction the subject slowly but surely allows the activity level of that part of the brain to fall. If this were so, then other parts of the brain, such as the anterior (forward) region, which directs attention, thought, and action, might gain temporary domination. The subject's attention, now pinch-hitting for his will, can be engaged by the hypnotist, whose suggestions are implanted as plans for future action. Later, these covert plans emerge when cued.

Reflex trance could work via a similar takeover of the posterior attentional system, which orients us to external signals. As the unexpected stimulus invades the abnormally unprotected networks of the brain stem, the susceptible subject's attention is instantly, unconsciously, and automatically disengaged. He loses his ability to orient; he loses contact with his surroundings. At the same time, the motor aspect of his startle response — also abnormally sensitive — is triggered and he jumps. It can happen to all of us, although usually to lesser degrees; when someone startles us, we "jump" as an integral part of our surprise reaction.

For centuries a shift in selective attention has been thought to be the mechanism of hypnosis. Now that we have a more detailed and brain-based theory of how selective attention works, it may be possible to specify the mechanisms that induce trance.

As we saw in Chapter 10, when we discussed attention in detail, it is also likely that our new knowledge of sleep-state control will help the effort to put hypnosis on a more solid scientific footing. For centuries the very term hypnosis, memorializing the Greek god of sleep, Hypnos, has signaled our awareness of a kinship between our spontaneous and induced brain-mind dissociations.

And indeed, sleep itself can be viewed as an automatism — an involuntary action that occurs without volition or neural stimulation. Becoming drowsy is akin to hypnosis; will and attention both fade as the activation level of the cortex falls. Once the activation falls below a certain point, the thalamus, that central filter that during waking blocks the cortex from being swamped with random signals, loses control, and the cortex is bombarded with powerful internal stimuli that further disorganize its activity. Now we are truly entranced — by sleep.

The behavior associated with Latah, or startle trance, is fascinating for several other reasons. The stream of foul-mouthed invectives uttered by the Malay strongly parallels that which occurs in Gilles de la Tourette's syndrome, in which compulsive swearing is often accompanied by involuntary arm flailing. These automatisms have a kinship with the dissociations of sleep: sleepwalking, sleeptalking, and the REM sleep behavior disorder are all characterized by automatic motor acts. All are unwilled and all are nonconscious.

JUMPING LUMBERJACKS!

The startle trance of Latah is not a quirk restricted to a particular Asian community. Similar traits are shared by an unusual group that is closer to home, the "Jumping Frenchmen" of northern Maine. These skittish lumberjacks are strikingly Latah-like, except that their startle behavior has no religious context whatever. Whether this curious trait is inherited or learned is not clear but it appears to provide social entertainment all week long. Tickling or surprise is again the stimulus; when a Jumping Frenchman is poked or ambushed, he immediately responds with a dramatic, almost convulsive jump. In its aftermath comes a stream of gutter speech and a trancelike dissociation of consciousness that promotes automatic obedience to the suggestions of onlookers.

Like reflex Latah, the behavior of the Jumping Frenchmen appears to involve a takeover of a brain-mind state that co-opts the posterior attention system. The orienting function of the brain stem and posterior network is jolted, causing the jump. Then a wave of excitation spreads rapidly upward, jamming the thalamus and momentarily disconnecting the anterior system. Thus released from voluntary control, restraint in the cortex is lost. The subjects become slavishly obedient to the suggestions of onlookers and emit a chorus of foul language as if some deep swearing center had become automatically activated.

The fact that the Jumping Frenchmen know they are subject to this behavior only makes their reactions worse. A young boy who knows that his older brother will scare him when he reaches the top of a dark staircase is scared even more when it happens. The anticipation heightens his response.

Both the Malaysian Latahs and the Jumping Frenchmen are isolated cultural groups, so it may be that religious beliefs and genetic inbreeding play roles. But the brain-mind state change that is seen in Latahs, Jumping Frenchmen, narcoleptics, and Tourette's patients evidences the common feature of increased sensitivity to stimuli. Sensory signals cause a sudden attentional shift. A motor automatism results. The usual chain of command involving consciousness, volition, and action is broken. Likewise, highly hypnotizable subjects who have been studied in our culture easily shift attention away from the outside world. In fact, these susceptible individuals are inclined to enter imaginative trancelike states whether or not they are in the presence of a hypnotist. This frequent and fluid state change has led to their characterization as lifelong fantasy addicts.

The most remarkable talent of highly hypnotizable subjects is their ability to perceive self-generated imagery of hallucinatory strength. For example, instead of calling up the outline or silhouette of an animal's head, as we are all able to do, these exceptional individuals can see the whole animal, embed it in a scene, and let the scene develop into a vivid movie. This natural talent for scenario projection — on the home movie screen of the individual's brain-mind — results in a pseudo-reality that most of us experience only when we dream. From a physiological viewpoint, it seems that highly hypnotizable people live closer to the edge of REM sleep than the rest of us do.

For obvious reasons, evolution has selected individuals who can maintain sharp boundaries between brain-mind states that involve shifts from external to internal attention. If one is to survive in any threatening environment, it is important to maintain alertness to danger. And in a task requiring sustained vigilance, such as stalking prey or flying a high-speed jet, the sudden intrusion of dream or fantasy images is extremely counterproductive.

We cross the Stage 1 boundary rapidly upon falling asleep and waking up. During this fleeting stage dreamlets may occur. We cross the boundary so quickly and automatically that we have little or no awareness of the curious mixtures of waking and dreaming consciousness that can occur. But we can prime our brain-minds, by suggestion, to slow this process down and perceive it, and with practice we can even achieve lucid dreaming. In both sleep onset and lucid dreaming, some aspects of waking have been drawn into dreaming. The result in both cases is a similarly dissociated state in which we regain some attentional and volitional control but continue to hallucinate. We can enjoy watching ourselves doing impossible things such as carefree flying and judgment-free sex. These altered states, for us, closely resemble the altered states of trance and hypnosis.

It should come as no surprise to learn that highly hypnotizable subjects, who flit about on the edge of dreaming when awake, also have a natural talent for lucid dreaming. They can approach the wake-dream state interface from either direction and hover there. Not surprisingly, either, these lucid dreamers tend to believe in the supernatural. It is a convenient and intriguing explanation for their states, which even the most critical brain-mind specialists have trouble understanding.

As easily as they can enhance certain stimuli, like inner vision, people who are highly hypnotizable can suppress others, like pain. This anesthesia switch is obviously useful if it can be controlled by the subject or at the suggestion of a hypnotist, as was the case with Dr. Drury's sailor and the Hodgkin's itch patients. My colleague David Spiegel has intriguing preliminary evidence that the electrical and metabolic activity of the cortex can be altered at will during hallucination. This promising lead could help provide hypnosis with the foundation in physiology that it needs to hold it safe in the harbor of science.

What can the housewife in Sheboygan hope to learn from the Latahs of Malaysia, the Jumping Frenchmen of Maine, and the neighbor afflicted with Tourette's syndrome or narcolepsy? Only that she shares with all of them built-in mechanisms for hypnosis-like state shifts, and that these mechanisms could be useful to her in aiding important functions (such as childbirth) if she could only learn to summon their common anesthetic properties. For most of us the mechanisms that trigger these states are so difficult to access that we are tempted to write off our more susceptible brethren as weirdos whom we are happy not to resemble. But this is a smug and shortsighted stance. As we now turn our attention to some garden-variety dissociations, let us thank our exceptional friends for helping us understand their talent for changing states and see what we can learn from their example.

SOMNAMBULISM AND SLEEPWALKING

Proneness to hallucination, mild addiction to fantasy, and the anesthesia-triggering ability of highly hypnotizable subjects put them at some clinical risk. While some observers see them as talented, others see them as so bizarre as to invite psychiatric diagnoses. Indeed, many controversies in psychiatry have pivoted on the way that this exceptional set of mind-brain state features has been interpreted. And the debate is not over. If anything, it seems to be heating up again, so it may be wise to quickly review some of the roots of this complex story.

In the second half of the last century, the neurology clinics of Paris and Vienna, as well as those of Madrid and Milan, were crowded with women who complained of amnesias, anesthesias, automatisms, and dreamy states of consciousness. The most famous center for the study of what was called Grand Hysteria was the clinic of Jean-Martin Charcot at the Salpêtrière hospital in Paris. The most dramatic event in Charcot's clinical repertoire was the induction of hypnotic trance.

The brain-mind state changes that Charcot and his illustrious team were able to induce included alterations in postural tone, reflex excitability, and attentiveness. These exotic physiological changes did much to rescue the curious behavior from the fringes of science. The father of hypnosis, the Austrian physician Franz Anton Mesmer (as in "mesmerized"), thought in the late 1700s that these state shifts were a reflection of animal magnetism. This concept, which had already been castigated by an official commission that included the lightning expert Benjamin Franklin, was replaced by Charcot's more scientific vocabulary.

But Charcot himself could not advance his theory beyond the important distinction that he drew, which was that abnormal function (which we would now see as an altered brain-mind state) was not necessarily the result of an anatomical lesion (fixed damage to the brain). Charcot's inability to specify exactly what he meant by "functional abnormality" left the door open to a wide variety of interpretations. The most famous of these was Sigmund Freud's development of the psychoanalytic theory. Psychoanalysis elaborated Charcot's own emphasis on thwarted sexual impulses. It also allowed some stray Mesmerists to sneak back into the center ring. As a colleague of mine has pointed out, magnets, batteries, and metal plates were once again in vogue.

Charcot coined the term "somnambulism" to describe the peculiar changes in posture, reflex response, and attentiveness that his patients exhibited, sometimes spontaneously and always when in hypnotically induced trance. Charcot's somnambulists were in a dissociative state with some features of waking and some features of sleep.

To help us understand this odd state we need only examine some details of modern somnambulism — plain old garden-variety sleepwalking. Many of us have done it, and most of us have seen it or one of its close relatives in our children. Today, the medical community calls such automatisms — sleeptalking, bed-wetting, tooth grinding, and night terrors — "parasomnias," to signal that these unusual sensorimotor behaviors occur within otherwise normal sleep. The two other major classes of sleep disorder are called *in*somnias (too little sleep) and *hyper*somnias (too much sleep).

Sleepwalking is a "functional" problem if ever there was one. Like Charcot, we would expect to see no structural lesion if we microscopically examined the brain of a sleepwalker. And we would expect to see no significant psychopathology in a mental status exam either. Sleepwalking is a slight but significant variation on a perfectly normal process of brain-mind state control.

When sleepwalking occurs in the sleep lab, the electrode recordings reveal a profound dissociation. One part of the sleepwalker's brain is asleep, another part is awake. Contrary to common sense, sleepwalkers are not acting out dreams. Their episodes do not occur during REM sleep. In fact, they occur during non-REM sleep. Sleepwalking is physiologically and behaviorally different from the REM-sleep behavior disorder demonstrated by José, the man who elbowed his wife while dreaming of driving his car. Instead of performing motor acts that conform to the hallucinations of a dream scenario, the sleepwalker performs motor acts that are appropriate to some realistic, if slightly misguided, external goal.

Part of the explanation is that during non-REM sleep, motor activity is not shut off. It is only reduced. Motor activity is not fully inhibited until REM sleep begins. In non-REM, there is still a low level of drive on the motor system (how else would we "roll over" in bed while we are asleep?). Note, too, that there is some level of brain activity during non-REM sleep as well; it is very diminished, but never "off." The goal that sleepwalkers are trying to reach is not fully conscious to them, but it is powerful enough to direct the body.

The amazing fact is that as the sleepwalker wanders, his eyes open, and sometimes he even converses with whoever is in the room. Parents of young children experience this frequently; their little sons or daughters may open their eyes and even reach for a hug when parents walk in during the middle of the night, yet they are still sleeping. In the lab, the EEG readings of sleepwalkers who are conversing with the attendants exhibit the same slow waves of normal Stage 4 sleep. This further supports the diagnosis that the upper part of the sleepwalker's brain, the cognitive part, is in deep sleep, while the lower part, the motor part, is awake. The sleepwalker is in two states at once.

In some cases, the sleepwalker has a completely unrealistic or potentially dangerous goal, like climbing out an upper-story window to a thin ledge. The old wives' tale that you shouldn't wake a sleepwalker is silly. You might not be *able* to wake him because his upper brain is in deep sleep. But the only reason a sleepwalker seems to jump in fright when awakened is because he has been startled from his state. The response is the same as that of someone who is seated at a desk concentrating, with his back to you, when you walk in and startled him: a reflexive jump, perhaps a flailing of the arms, and a moment of anger at the jolt. More commonly, a sleepwalker is simply headed for the bathroom, but because his maps are mixed up, he ends up in the living room or the kitchen. I myself was quite capable, when a young man, of sleepwalking down a full flight of stairs, opening the front door, and urinating in the rose garden.

Children are particularly prone to this form of dissociation, probably because they sleep so much more deeply. This has led to the theory that all the parasomnias are "disorders of arousal." A stimulus like a full bladder is sufficient to arouse an older person from sleep. When we say to the parent of a bed-wetter or a sleep-walker, "Just be patient, your child will grow out of it," it's true. Maturation, in this case, is the loss of an entirely normal brain-mind function — a dissociation.

We lose other brain-mind functions in mid-life or late life, such as the ability to enter Stage 4 sleep. Many older folks never sleep deeply, and if they would stop worrying about it, it would have no affect on their health. Yet our capacity to grow out of one problem is matched — or even exceeded — by our capacity to grow into another one. One elderly patient of mine said that, for her, old age was a problem because she had more time in which to do less. By that she meant that her diminished sleep need — reflected in her shorter and shallower epochs of sleep — was not balanced by an increase in energy or enthusiasm for work or pleasure to fill the extra waking hours. Society had not provided her with diverting or satisfying alternatives to the sense of useless boredom that was the real pain of her insomnia. In the face of a shrunken and less elastic brain, the only adaptive response older people can take comfort in is to alter the way the information in their brain-mind is processed. That kind of reframing of mental content is called wisdom.

THE TAPE-RECORDER CURE

Sleeptalking is an amusing variation on the theme of dissociation. Stories about nocturnal monologues and dialogues usually provoke mirth and mild embarrassment. Not all is innocent fun, however; damaging confessions can be extracted by spouses suspicious of hanky-panky, although these admissions would never hold up in court because they are collected without the subject's conscious compliance and because the subject is too prone to the suggestions made by the midnight interviewer.

Until recently, it was common for psychiatrists to assume that all sleep disorders were manifestations of unconscious motivation. And, indeed, a man who finds himself snacking from his icebox while half asleep at 1:00 A.M. may do well to wonder what this behavior suggests. For the vast majority of people with sleep disorders, however, there is no psychological undercurrent. Their eccentricities are purely the result of dissociation.

Consider the case of Frank Morewill. Frank was a hardworking and handsome apprentice electrician who had just married his high school sweetheart. He slept enviably well but was horrified to learn from his young bride that — like the Latahs, the Jumping Frenchmen, and the Tourette's patients — he had a foul tongue that led a life of its own when he was asleep.

The young wife was not shocked. She knew all those words and accepted the obvious fact that Frank knew them too. If his sleep-cursing awakened her, all she needed to do was give him a poke to get him to roll over, and peace reigned again in their bedroom. But Frank was worried about his going on a swearing binge during a night when his in-laws were guests in the adjacent bedroom. They would think their daughter had married a monster.

When I met Frank, I was just beginning to realize how much I and my patients could learn about sleep behavior without resorting to a sleep lab. So I asked Frank, "Why not simply tape-record the swearing and have your wife enter the date and time of each occurrence?" A $50 hand-held tape recorder is much cheaper than a $10,000 polygraph and has a much wider variety of uses.

So Frank went to the local gadget shop and picked up a voice-activated recorder that he placed on his bedside table. One month later he returned to see me, clutching his tape recorder and his sleep chart. He was beaming. I didn't know what to anticipate from his broad smile.

"This tape recorder is wonderful!" he exclaimed. "Since you prescribed it, I haven't sworn at all."

I must confess that while I was pleased that he was pleased, I was a bit lost. Furthermore, I hadn't "prescribed" anything. Then it hit me. I had unwittingly used the power of suggestion on Frank. He had responded positively to the social pressure of a monitoring device, and his view that this was my "prescription" added legitimacy to the notion. I didn't want to negate this desirable placebo effect, so I suggested that, just to be on the safe side, he keep the tape recorder at his beside for another month and call me if he had anything to report. "I'm cured," he said confidently, and sure enough, he never called me again.

Since being educated by Frank, I have seen four other cases of parasomnia that were cured by the presence of a monitoring device.

THE PLACEBO EFFECT

We all expect to be helped by a doctor. Even the medical profession's current fall from grace doesn't seem to change the deep drive toward health and optimism that prompts us to seek help. It is so strong in us that even a disenchanted patient is likely to come away feeling better.

This perverse but welcome phenomenon is called the placebo effect. "Placebo" in Latin means "I shall please." It is a very powerful force accounting for between one-third and two-thirds of the perceived benefits of medical care. The effect is so powerful it now forms the basis for testing new treatment modalities. New drugs cannot be presented to the FDA for approval until they have been tested against a control group — people who are given what they believe to be a new cure but in reality is only a sugar pill. Any new treatment must overcome the uphill battle of proving that it provides a significant improvement in outcome statistics over those obtained with sugar tablets.

How should we think about this phenomenon and what should the doctor and the patient do about it? One response that I would not recommend is to devalue it by saying it's not "real" medicine. That's like discounting hypnosis because it involves suggestion. The worst thing of all would be to suppose that the placebo effect is no effect at all. We are in danger of that scientific mistake when we call it "nonspecific" or even "psychological," implying it is "nothing but." If a placebo works, it works — somehow. And our job as scientific humanists is to find out how. Meanwhile let us prescribe, take, and enjoy the benefits of as many placebos as we can find, while admitting our ignorance as to how such a harmless and inexpensive medicine can be so effective. Another mistake would be to try to get rid of it. You can't kill hope.

LEARNING FROM DELIA

My friend Delia has taught me more than Charcot, Freud, and Mesmer put together about the nature of brain-mind states and how they can be used to benefit health and the deep enjoyment of life. Nothing is alien to Delia. On the contrary, she sees even her sometimes terrifying dreams and her painfully depressed states of waking as both instructive and inspirational. Although she is more fatalistic than I would care to be, she is also truer to herself than I would dare to be. As a result, she is able to respond positively to a wide variety of psychological, physiological, and spiritual issues.

We have already seen how Delia uses her rich and abundant dream life as an existential theater — to be enjoyed or suffered, but in any case accepted, attended to, and even celebrated. She goes to bed looking forward to dreaming and she wakes up the wiser for having dreamed. Her dream journal is a treasure trove of her psychic experience, some of which she has been good enough to share with us. While most of us will never match Delia on the scales of dream exoticism or amount of recall, we can all learn to increase our awareness of dreaming and to increase the intensity and quality of our dream experience.

Delia is also daringly experimental when given the chance to increase either her psychic experience or her knowledge about it. She has slept in the sleep lab and been awakened during REM sleep for dream reports. She also has used my lab's new home-based REM detector, the Nightcap, which enables her to chart her sleep signals on a personal computer positioned beside her bed. Delia uses the Nightcap to increase her access to dreams and has discovered, just as Swedenborg did, that after she has been sleep-deprived her dreams become more intense and more inclusive of themes that themes that are important to her, like relationships with people she loves or the venerated figures from her religious world. One of Delia's most exotic experiments with dreaming is the cultivation of lucidity or dream consciousness. With practice, she has been able to gain awareness that she is dreaming while she is dreaming. In so doing she can shape her dream life in forms that she seeks, like flying (without a balloon) and enjoying sex (even with forbidden partners). Thus she incorporates the science of dreaming into her intellectual growth and her own particular view of the world and the cosmos. Delia said it herself — she is definitely New Age.

But Delia is not immune to the stresses of modern life. Far from it. She is typical of the 1990s city dweller, with a high-pressure job and lifestyle. For Delia, the luxury of dropping out is just not an option. So when she gets up early and commutes to her office, she plays a relaxation instructional tape on her car stereo. This holds her brain-mind in a relatively peaceful state as the traffic whizzes, honks, and halts around her. And when her boss gives her more work than three of her could complete in a day, she calls on her inner voice to reassure herself — and her boss — that she will do her best but that she cannot do the impossible.

When work stress raises its voice to a screaming pitch, Delia does drop out, but only by changing state. Not by quitting. She can close her eyes, sit still, and enter a trancelike meditative state in seconds. Twenty minutes of emergency meditation can also rescue her from social embarrassment when she finds herself with people who are insensitive or ungiving. Instead of losing her temper — and her self-respect — she beats a strategic retreat to her meditative haven, from which she emerges refreshed and armed with both distance and a calmer perspective.

Delia's health has been plagued by the usual host of minor problems, and some major ones, too. When she needs to consult professionals — like dentists and doctors — she does so comfortably, knowing that she can control both the inevitable discomfort of diagnosis and treatment, and the sometimes alarming messages these encounters can deliver.

Although as prone to anxiety about her health as we all are, Delia manages her anxiety actively by letting her insight about its natural, instinctual nature help her find equally natural channels of relief. One is the meditative practice already mentioned. Another is sleep. And still another is exercise. So far she has not yet turned to formal hypnosis, but if she needed it, she would not hesitate to try it. And because she is already so talented and so practiced at state change, she believes that even deep trance would not be beyond her reach.

And none of these nostrums precludes her use of dreams to create a model of her life history, her current crisis, and her options for the future. These are the concerns of traditional psychotherapy, which can also flourish in the rich atmosphere of the new brain-mind paradigm. Delia's conscious states are thus both a blueprint and a proving ground for life change.

CHAPTER 15

The Last Resort: Using Drugs to Change Your State

T HE BRAIN-MIND has the ability to heal itself by changing states. You can harness this power to improve your health — both mental and physical — by voluntarily altering your state of being. Some people, however, fall prey to excessive stress, addiction, disease, and the simple long-term death of brain cells. Drugs are often helpful in changing the brain-mind states of these people, the Bertals of the world, whom we so readily label as "abnormal." And with the advent of new cure-alls like Prozac, even very normal folk are likely to be offered potent state-altering medication.

There is no doubt that the development of drugs that interact with the brain-mind's chemical system is the most important advance in the history of modern psychiatry. Drugs are fundamental to man's attempts to correct such debilitating disorders as schizophrenia, mania, and depression, not to mention diseases that can ruin the brain, such as tumors, infections, diabetes, and meningitis. Drugs make it possible to alter the altered states of the mentally ill. If we add to the list vitamins such as thiamine and niacin, which can often cure the organic psychoses brought on by alcohol and drug dependency, there can be no doubt that chemistry has revolutionized our understanding of mental illness and our capacity to treat it.

Why, then, wouldn't an intelligent person consider pharmacology to be his best treatment option? Shouldn't the most powerful tool for changing the state of the brain-mind in a desirable direction be a drug? In most cases the answer is "Yes, but . . ." The use of a drug can be as problematic as it is preemptive. For that reason I myself prescribe drugs reluctantly and prefer in as many cases as possible to manipulate a patient's chemistry by natural means.

By widely deploying the set of chemicals that regulate our brains and bodies — most importantly, norepinephrine, serotonin, and acetylcholine — nature has made our job both simple and impossibly difficult. When we give any drug that is aimed at the brain-mind, we cannot avoid hitting the whole body and all its many physiological control systems. We must acknowledge the risk of both unspecific and undesirable consequences — "side effects" — as well as dynamic adaptations of the affected system: addiction and habituation.

We must also face the fact that almost none of the chemicals we use today as drugs are made by the body. For example, there is no clearly effective natural sedative. We also know that our drug treatments are not only unnatural, they are not even aimed at the deepest level of biological mechanism: the gene. Finally there is a host of drug abuses to consider, ranging from the personal, through the professional and commercial, to the more broadly social.

Drugs are a powerful aid to changing the brain-mind states of the mentally ill, but we must use them with appropriate caution.

One afternoon, when I was a third-year medical student and just beginning my obstetrics rotation at the Boston Lying-In Hospital, I came home with a dreadful head cold. My sinuses and upper respiratory passages were so congested I felt as clogged as a stopped drain. Any sensible person would have thrown in the towel, called in sick, and crawled into bed. But my curiosity about the birthing process and a sense of responsibility toward my fellow students and future patients urged me not to miss a day of this important learning experience.

To relieve my symptoms, a roommate recommended that I take one of his antihistamine pills. He said they had worked wonders on his recent cold. In the medicine cabinet of the house we shared I found the bottle — labeled Phenergan, 25 mg. — and popped a pill. Within a few hours, and before I could really say whether my cold symptoms were better or not, I began to have a strange new set of sensations throughout my body. They persisted for the next two days, during which I assisted in four uncomplicated deliveries, one cesarean section, and one emergency operation for an ectopic pregnancy.

I found it amazing that no one noticed anything unusual about me. Apparently I looked and acted sufficiently normal to pass for me — with a head cold. But from my vantage point I felt removed from the world around me. I felt cut off, sensorially and psychically insulated in a fuzzy cocoon that had spun itself around me. What was going on?

The answer would only come a year or so later, when it was shown that Phenergan, in addition to being an antihistamine, was also a major tranquilizer, from the same chemical family as the chlorpromazine we had prescribed for Bertal at The Psycho. As was the case with chlorpromazine, Phenergan's tranquilizing effects were discovered only by accident after it had been tried out as a cold remedy. These two drugs, it was found, had a wide variety of effects because, in addition to blocking histamine, they also blocked the action of dopamine, another amine that plays a role in modulating the brain. A dopamine deficiency causes Parkinson's disease. When dopamine is actively blocked in a healthy individual, that person can actually undergo Parkinson-like experiences. And because the drugs also interfere with the action of acetylcholine, they may cause dryness of the mouth, blurred vision, and dizziness. The sensation I felt was strong, distinctive, and weird. I have no doubt that I changed state because I had taken a pill that altered the balance of the natural state-control chemicals in my brain.

THE BODY'S DRUGS AND MAN'S INTERFERENCE

To understand why drugs are both effective and problematic, it helps to know a little about how the body's key chemicals carry out their duties. My own favorite molecule, acetylcholine, is responsible for an amazing array of functions. It not only battles with the amines for daily control over my brain-mind states, it can slow my heart, make every muscle in my body twitch, constrict the pupils of my eyes, make me salivate, or cause me to blush. This one molecule is utilized by practically every cell in the body for one purpose or another. If it could only find its way into my brain stem, when administered from outside, without going everywhere else — but of course it can't.

In each duty, acetylcholine works by conveying messages between nerve cells. The endings of adjacent nerve cells are separated by a tiny space called the synapse. Like the outstretched fingers of God and Man painted by Michelangelo on the ceiling of the Sistine Chapel, the nerve endings extend to meet each other but don't quite touch. When one nerve cell needs to communicate with the next, it squirts a few acetylcholine molecules out of the end of its finger and they ferry the information across the synapse to the tip of the second nerve cell.

When the molecules reach the other side, they are locked into place by receptors, special structures on the neuron's membrane that deform slightly to "grasp" the molecules. It's as if a ferryboat left the end of a dock on one side of a river, crossed the water, then found an open slip on a dock on the other side; if there are no suitable openings when the ship arrives, the receptor cells shove a few boats apart from each other to make room. Or not. The receptor cells must decide whether to accept the messenger boat and lock it in, or refuse it and keep it adrift.

Because acetylcholine and other key chemicals affect so many functions, it is nearly impossible to localize their action to a single system. Imagine that I wanted to increase the amount of acetylcholine available to my muscles (as would be the case if I had the muscle-weakness disease called myasthenia gravis). How could I get a drug to help the acetylcholine in my muscles without it also going to my heart or my eyes? I couldn't. Once the drug has entered my bloodstream it can go almost anywhere in my body.

The "almost" is important because the one place it might actually have the most trouble reaching is the brain. The brain is so important that it is protected from invasion by the so-called blood-brain barrier. Though not fully understood, the blood-brain barrier is effectively a membrane that surrounds the brain. All blood vessels feeding the brain must pass through it, and at each crossing point unwanted molecules are turned back by physical, chemical, or electrical means. Only a few molecules that circulate in the blood are admitted freely, such as oxygen and sugar. Most molecules, including some that we would very much like to see get to the brain, are excluded.

The net result is trouble for pharmacological assaults on the brain-mind. Most medicinal drugs that are ingested or injected will go to virtually every cell outside the brain but will be prevented from reaching the brain. If the brain is our target, we are very likely to miss it — while inadvertently hitting everything else. Not surprisingly, most recreational drugs get through the blood-brain barrier easily. That's why they are so popular and so dangerous.

Because the body uses acetylcholine to transact so much of its business, it has developed some chemical tricks to improve and regulate the specificity of its action. The body regulates acetylcholine with an enzyme called cholinesterase. The enzyme, in the synapse, chews up acetylcholine and spits it out in little pieces on contact. In this way, cholinesterase interrupts and shuts off signals as rapidly as they are generated, which is normal and necessary. In the time it has taken me to write this sentence, I have made thousands of minute hand and finger movements, each of which depended on the prompt release and prompt breakdown of millions of acetylcholine molecules to coordinate the tiny muscles in my hand.

The upshot is that if I were to inject acetylcholine into my bloodstream (or into my brain stem, if that were somehow possible) it would be effective for at most one second, after which every one of the millions of molecules I injected would be chewed up! That's why my colleague Roberto and his mates (Chapter 4) injected carbachol, a man-made chemical, into the brains of cats that were awake to switch them to REM sleep and keep them there. Carbachol mimics the action of acetylcholine but cannot be chewed up by cholinesterase.

The problem with using synthetic chemicals such as carbachol for clinical treatments is that they have a vast set of side effects that may take years to emerge and fully understand. That's why pharmacology is, for me, a last resort. And that's why I am a reluctant chemist. When it comes to treating brain-mind state disorders, the best approach is preventive maintenance. The best person to create an effective preventive maintenance program for your brain-mind is you.

The body regulates chemical signaling in another ingenious way. Neurons always try to maintain a moderate number of receptor sites — open slips — on their membranes so that when a signal first comes in it can quickly be received. The incoming acetylcholine molecules fill the empty receptor slips. If, as the slips fill, the docks continue to be bombarded with molecules, the neuron reconfigures itself so no more slips are available. It literally changes the shape of the cell membrane so there are no more open receptor sites. In the presence of a high concentration of an incoming molecule, the receptor sites decrease in number. This process is called "down-regulation." We must admire nature's economy: because there is so much transmitter available, there is no need for so many receptors to ensure that messages will get through. Each neuron varies the availability of receptors according to local conditions.

This process of adaptation, however, results in habituation. When we continually use drugs that affect the brain-mind, the neurons get used to having so much of the chemical around, and the receptor sites remain shut down. The neuron becomes insensitive to the messengers that are shouting at dock's edge to be let in. Within a few days, most drugs become less effective, so we need more of them to accomplish the same effect. Notice that *habituation* is the same word we used to describe the rapid adaptation of our brain-minds to repeated stimuli when we discussed the startle reflex. When I tried to scare my office-mate a second time, and a third, he didn't jump; he learned cognitively that there was no threat. He had become habituated. The same learning occurs with drug usage, albeit at the cellular level.

Our nonconscious brain-minds are much smarter than we think. If we do use a medicinal or recreational drug, we should respect the long-term habituation process. The smart move is for consciousness to order frequent abstention from drugs, so that the nonconscious brain-mind can restore its sensitivity.

Sensitivity, so to speak, is restored by another ingenious process. When the river becomes jammed with acetylcholine molecules that cannot find receptor sites, the neuron sending the acetylcholine slows down its output and eventually stops. This is evidence again of nature's economy; we don't need the stuff, so we don't make any more.

There is one drawback to this process. If the neural network suddenly decides it needs to receive more messages, the neurons that have stopped producing acetylcholine will not be ready to re-supply the molecules. It takes time to get the acetylcholine factory cranked up to full production. Depending on the type of neurons involved, the lag can be minutes, hours, days, or even weeks. As a result, the neurons on the receiving end are crying out for messengers but aren't getting any. This is called withdrawal. It's a normal and unnoticeable phenomenon that occurs after everyday actions. But it can be much more extreme when a drug is used and dosage and length of use reach excessive levels.

There is one way for the individual in withdrawal to stop the anguish: give the desperate receptor cells a quick shot of the chemical they're looking for. Take another pill, swig another drink, insert another syringe. What has become of the person in this cycle? Unbeknownst to his conscious brain-mind, the neural networks in his nonconscious brain-mind have undergone a major change in state. Their only desire is to stabilize their distress by finding the magic missing molecule: the drug. Adaptation, habituation, dependence, addiction, and withdrawal — a sequence that, in one way or another, is triggered every time someone alters the dynamics of the metabolism that normally regulates the neurotransmitters sending messages between cells. This vicious cycle is yet another reason why I am a reluctant chemist.

There is nothing more unsatisfying to me than treating, with a drug, a disorder that has been created by another drug. But so common are the side effects of brain-mind chemicals that it is the rule, rather than the exception, to need not one drug but two, or three, or even four to balance the tilted brain-mind and body. And so strong is the adaptation-habituated-addiction sequence that even drug withdrawals often have to be covered with other drugs.

This deleterious cycle results in part because brain-mind states reflect a constantly negotiated settlement between opposing forces: waking and REM sleep; excitation and inhibition; ergotropic and trophotropic; aminergic and cholinergic. If the balance of these reciprocal systems is tipped in one direction, a reactive and corrective change takes place in the opposite direction.

The problem is that a chemically induced correction can often lead to a backlash; the pendulum is swung too far in the opposite direction. A classic example is the overly effective reversal of depression by a drug that then launches the patient into mania. Another is the suppression of aggressive behavior with drugs that, as a side effect, turn off REM sleep; as we've seen, REM sleep fights back, and in this case breaks through as terrifying nightmares.

The point is obvious: every shift in the balance of a brain-mind system triggers a reactive shift. It's a twist on Newton's second law: every brain-mind action has an equal and opposite reaction. The give-and-take of ergotropic and trophotropic drives is an integral part of our nonconscious brain-minds. It is this ability to oscillate between such different states as waking and dreaming that confers a large measure of our adaptive flexibility, and as such it is the very fulcrum of the lever of our health.

The wake-dream oscillations are controlled by catalysts. Vitamins are the catalysts of brain-mind chemistry. Catalysts are like the activity directors on cruise ships — they facilitate the action but do not participate. Catalysts are molecules that are essential for metabolism to proceed but are not themselves used up in the reactions they incite. Thiamine (vitamin B_1) and riboflavin (vitamin B_2) are two examples. Their presence is required for the enzymes in nerve cells to crank out neurotransmitters.

Our bodies cannot make vitamins. We must consume them in our diet. And now that their molecular structures are well known, it is very difficult to avoid them. They are added to food during the manufacturing process. Just take a look at a cereal box in your kitchen and you will realize that the minimum daily requirement of many vitamins is consumed by most of us long before we reach for that bottle of vitamin pills.

RECOVERING FROM SKID ROW

Now that we understand how the body's key chemicals carry out their duties, and how drugs can interrupt or tip the balance of these processes, we can apply our knowledge to solving problems of brain-mind states. In keeping with the tenets of scientific humanism, I will present three cases that show how drugs are most effectively used as bridges to more natural and permanent cures. The three cases present very different disorders of the brain-mind state system and illustrate the range of mental illnesses that can be first arrested with drugs, then treated in the long term with voluntary control of states.

New York City is famous for many landmarks. One small section of town, The Bowery, has become legendary as the gathering place for the city's winos. It is the prototypical skid row. On the south side of Boston, skid row is found along Washington Street, under the "el" (the elevated subway). That's where Jerry Gross spent much of his time. Jerry had bounced from one job to another and couldn't seem to hang on to his money. Solace for his woes took the form of a drink, which served primarily to further deplete his already thin wallet.

Jerry woke up one morning on the grass of Boston Common, where he had passed out in drunken stupor the night before with other alcohol addicts of the city. Jerry had become a drunk. It made him mad. Mad at the world. So mad he began to mumble about it to the imaginary friend who tagged along beside him as he wandered up and down Washington Street. So mad he ranted and raved about it to people who hurriedly passed him by. So mad he took a drink. And another. Until his money ran out, which made him madder still. He boldly approached people for money, shouting at whoever turned him down. He never got much, perhaps a rare handful of change, so food became out of the question. Who wanted food? What he needed to feel better was a drink. And the cheaper the booze the better.

Jerry roamed and raved and panhandled and drank, day after day, week after week. He slept in doorways. He urinated in alleys. His arms and legs began to swell, and some nights, after sleeping on the hard ground, he couldn't move his body to get up. When he did get up, he would get into people's faces, pressing his smelly, famished body against them until they gave him a coin or shoved him away. Until the cops caught up with him and thrust him into the medical ward of Boston City Hospital.

Everyone in the hospital admitting room could tell Jerry was an alcoholic. But the doctors knew what his most immediate medical problem was: beriberi. This disease wreaks havoc on the nervous system and ultimately results in paralysis and swelling of the body. It results from thiamine deficiency. About the only way to become thiamine deficient in the modern world is to become a dietary dropout — to abandon food in favor of a drug, in Jerry's case, alcohol. After six weeks or so of this behavior, the brain-mind is not only permanently intoxicated, it is on the edge of organic psychosis. When awake, Jerry would ramble on to his imaginary friend. He was living in a dream world, quite literally. His waking psychosis, his visions, his disorientation and confabulation and memory loss, were similar to Delia's dream visions, her dream psychosis. And the chemical cause was parallel; Delia's sleeping brain is deprived of amines, enabling acetylcholine to take over and cause her to dream. Jerry's vitamin-starved brain could no longer produce any amines, and so his visions wandered with him up Washington Street.

The organic mental syndrome of skid row is often called Korsakoff's psychosis, not because that august Russian neurologist drank too much vodka, but because he described the syndrome and recognized it to be a physical consequence of alcohol abuse. When Korsakoff's psychosis is associated with paralysis of the eye muscles and a limitation of outward gaze, the larger and far graver picture is called Wernicke's encephalopathy.

Budding neurologists (and you qualify if you've read this far) will be interested to note that the part of the brain that is most sensitive to thiamine deficiency is the brain stem, which controls our states. As Jerry moved inexorably toward Korsakoff-Wernicke bedlam, he could no longer enter REM sleep and he stopped dreaming. In attempting a correction, his waking brain-mind state had swung too far in the opposite direction, and it assumed the properties of dreaming around the clock. What Jerry's nonconscious brain-mind needed — I'm sorry to say, some weeks before the police dragged him into the hospital — was shots of vitamin B_1 instead of the shots of cheap wine he consciously craved.

Surely a more significant triumph would be to prevent alcoholism altogether. As we contemplate what is required to achieve that goal we may gain further understanding of why it is so important — and why it is so difficult — to be a reluctant chemist.

Here, nonetheless, is a real cure for a curious, life-threatening psychiatric disorder. No wonder Linus Pauling and other sophisticated scientists have pushed B-vitamin therapy so hard against other serious disorders, such as schizophrenia.

Unfortunately, Jerry had passed the point at which vitamins — and abstinence — would have corrected his problem. As we will see shortly, he had to undergo a much more frightening brain-mind state change before he was able to wander onto the road to recovery.

How is the brain-mind state change affected by alcohol? Why is alcohol so irresistible? Most casual drinkers would argue that alcohol promotes relaxation, communication, and a sense of wellbeing. Alcohol does so by putting just enough of our neurons into just enough of a slump to allow others to emerge from the shadow of inhibition. Intoxication is definitely the right word for even the mildest effects of alcohol. We are actually giving ourselves a drug that could, if the dose were increased, cause sleep, stupor, coma, and even anesthesia as more and more neurons are put out of commission.

Getting high on alcohol or other recreational chemicals often means feeling elated — or at least less depressed than usual. So we have the paradox of a chemical that is just as much an anxiety breaker (a depressant) as it is an energizer (an antidepressant). By reducing behavioral inhibitions, alcohol promotes emotional expression. The personal interaction at a high-spirited cocktail party often moves from jollity (and joking) to elation (and self-revelation) to affection (and intimacy) to erotic stimulation (and sexual attraction).

If we could keep our conscious brain-mind on track, we could control the dose and kind of alcohol we use to get the perceived benefits without the liabilities. The problem is that we cannot control our intake because our good judgment is ruined as our inhibitions are released. Inappropriate behavior, gregariousness, even anger may set in as our bodies try to rid themselves of the self-administered drug.

Alcohol is one of the worst depressant drugs we can take because the body breaks alcohol down into by-products that are toxic. That middle-of-the-night awakening to a sick feeling occurs because the liver is busy knocking hydrogen off the ethanol molecules and turning them into formaldehyde — a substance commonly used for embalming. To say "I'm pickled" is thus not entirely metaphorical.

By 3:00 A.M. after an evening of carousing, the employees of your brain stem are awash in toxins. They are so unhappy they go on sleep strike. They refuse to create REM sleep until management improves the working conditions. But management, deprived of REM sleep, is in no position to think clearly. The alcohol and its by-products prevent the cholinergic system from discharging acetylcholine in the uninhibited way that it does during REM sleep. After a prolonged period of REM suppression it seems that the cholinergic system is under a marked increase in pressure.

The increase in pressure throws the brain-mind system out of balance. It can't control itself anymore, and the pendulum oscillates wildly. Alcoholics are brought to the hospital because their brain-minds are no longer capable of managing even the alcohol-seeking behavior. Like Jerry, they are found wandering aimlessly about, confused, disoriented, unable to remember, confabulating, and — the last straw — hallucinating.

These problems arise not because REM sleep is lost, but because it is suppressed. Researchers have been able to study the difference thanks to new antidepressant drugs like nialamide, which eliminate REM sleep without dire consequence. The function of REM sleep is to give the amines a rest, so they can rejuvenate. The new drugs rejuvenate the amines directly, so there is no need for REM sleep. The function of REM sleep is replaced. Alcohol suppresses REM sleep — it does not allow the amines to rest, and it does not boost them either. Recall that, in a healthy person, when REM sleep is lost for a night or two it is paid back with interest on subsequent nights. In an alcoholic, constant suppression of REM sleep causes the tension in the cholinergic system to mount until REM sleep comes crashing through, in the form of hallucinations.

The alcoholic who has reached this stage is in a dangerous downward spiral. The only way to break it is to abstain from alcohol, so the brain-mind can rid itself of the toxins. During withdrawal, the brain-mind oscillates out of control, and the spring-loaded cholinergic system, after such long suppression, takes over. Sleep is completely dominated by REM periods, and terrifying hallucinations occur at random. This acute payback, and the tremulousness it causes, are known as delirium tremens — the DTs, the shakes, or rum fits.

The fact that this delirium has all the formal features of normal dreaming, together with the increase in REM sleep that is observed as withdrawal proceeds, tempts us to speculate that the psychosis itself is a REM-like state. Unlike Delia's dream delirium — a REM psychosis confined to sleep — the DT psychosis occurs in a dissociated fashion, during waking. The fact that seizures may occur also invites comparison with the nearly epileptic nature of neuronal discharge that is normally confined to REM sleep.

Treating a patient who has DTs is itself a harrowing experience. I know because I had to see Jerry through this travail. Jerry's episodes of DT mania, and those of others I have helped, are among the most memorable experiences of my medical adventures. Many of these patients had other life-threatening illness, too, including raging cases of tuberculosis acquired due to exposure, poor diet, and poor sleep.

It was a hot, humid morning in August when the police brought Jerry into Boston City Hospital. His brain-mind could no longer regulate even his basic bodily functions. Remember those lab rats which, after six weeks of REM deprivation, were no longer able to maintain the most fundamental bodily housekeeping tasks, and died? Jerry was close to the same demise. The next two days were scorchers. Jerry ranted around the ward, then fell asleep only to wake up screaming from nightmares. In the hot afternoon of the third day, his body oscillated out of control. His temperature soared to 106°F. At 108°F brain cells die en masse. Jerry's brain was about to fry. We ran for the ice packs and thrust him into a tub of freezing water. His temperature plummeted to 88°F, close to the point of fatal hypothermia. So we warmed him, and he immediately overheated like a car engine. Back to the ice.

Each cycle his blood pressure skyrocketed, then nosedived, at some points bottoming out in the 60s; at a blood pressure of 60 even, the blood vessels can no longer diffuse enough oxygen into the brain, causing a loss of consciousness and coma. The neurotransmitters — the norepinephrine and acetylcholine that regulate the ergotropic and trophotropic divisions of the autonomic nervous systems that control body temperature and blood pressure — could not coordinate themselves. And all the while Jerry had horrifying waking REM hallucinations: legions of bugs crawled up the walls in Jerry's visions and all over his body. We knew we had to stabilize the pendulum soon, because after twenty-four hours of this autonomic tornado Jerry's kidneys would shut down, his liver would fold up, and his heart would just stop. He would die of brain-mind state control failure. Just like a rat. We had lost other drunks in the same way.

Luckily — and luck doesn't hurt in these cases — Jerry's mind and body responded to our efforts, and he stabilized. He remained in the hospital for three weeks. We treated him with vitamins to restore his brain function and with tranquilizers to keep his REM-sleep rebound within tolerable limits.

As his mind cleared and he began eating a normal diet, Jerry expressed the bravado that is typical of the recovering alcoholic. He had seen the light, he said. He would never drink again. He was cured and he was forever grateful to us. But we knew that only if he got hooked up with Alcoholics Anonymous to assure his abstinence would he be able to avoid a relapse to the toxic state in which we had found him. And only once solidly sober could Jerry begin to benefit from the sorts of voluntary brain-mind state control procedures that Delia has used so effectively.

BEATING INSOMNIA

The physiological chaos of DTs proves that a brain-mind state disorder can be fatal, without there being any disease in the brain. Jerry Gross's problem was an entirely functional organic disorder. There is nothing either imaginary or nonorganic about a functional disorder. As in sleep deprivation, sudden infant death syndrome, and Voodoo Death, vital functions can be so deranged as to cease functioning. Indeed, perhaps all death is the result of some functional disorder.

I emphasize this point to counter the pernicious tendency of psychoanalysis to foster the notion of "functional psychoses," implying that these derangements are only psychological, not organic. For Freud, these include schizophrenia and manic depression. For most of this century, this notion led to an exclusive emphasis on psychodynamic factors as causal in schizophrenia and to the now universally discredited notion that such major disturbances can be reversed by psychotherapy alone. Far more subtle and far more difficult to correct today, however, is the equally fatuous idea that the so-called psychosomatic complaints of many patients in hospital outpatient clinics are "all in the mind" — as if anything could be in the mind without being every bit as much in the brain.

Even at its lunatic peak in the 1960s, psychoanalysis did not offer to treat the DTs with conversation. However, on Park Avenue and in Beverly Hills some Freudians were still offering drunks the talking cure.

Like a brain-mind system that overcorrects itself, the psychiatric pendulum in recent years has swung too far in the opposite direction, toward overuse of drugs. Often when I address a large medical audience, I am aware of an impatient toleration of my views. The doctors wait out my sermon about scientific humanism, then, as if it passed right through their skulls, ask which drugs I prescribe for insomnia, depression, and schizophrenia. My answer is that I have experimented with practically all the usual agents and have had my share of success and problems with each of them.

As much as possible, I try to use drugs only to help the patient move as quickly as possible to a new state of mind. With new perspective and a sense of control, he can then begin to build up his ultimate reliance on physiology and psychology, without chemical aid.

This plan works not only for people, like Jerry, with extreme problems, but for all of us who have bouts with less dramatic, but still debilitating, brain-mind disorders. Which brings us to our second case, that of Miranda Prospero.

Miranda was a lovely young woman who had been unable to sleep since she had arrived in Boston to attend a high-powered graduate school. Despite her constant anxiety she had done outstanding academic work and had moved into a challenging job. According to the psychiatrist who referred her to me, all she needed was a well-chosen sedative and she would be fine. She was said to be happily married. She came from a large, supportive family. And she had her career wagon hooked to the stars. Unfortunately, she rarely stopped working, and when she did she couldn't stop thinking about work, so she couldn't sleep. One part of her cortex was telling her "You are tired," but another part was telling her "You've got to keep processing," and it called on the brain stem to continually send up norepinephrine to support the command. Miranda was voluntarily denying her sleep state by consciously remaining fixed on work. She was pushing her system beyond its limits, and soon enough she would collapse.

This advance billing prepared me for a hard-driving, unreflective overachiever, and before our first meeting I thought to myself, "I bet I will never get anywhere with this lady." My anticipation could not have been more wrong. My colleague failed to mention that Miranda Prospero was also very beautiful, caring, and sensitive. Miranda was a bionic woman all right, but one who whistled in the dark, and who was ready to reflect, to learn more about herself, and to change her brain-mind little by little so that, ultimately, she would not need sleeping pills.

In the three years since Miranda first consulted me, startling revelations have occurred during our dialogue and dramatic changes have taken place in her life. She has remembered scenes from her childhood when her father, a naval officer, beat her and her sisters. She has given up the entirely irrational idea that her nose, broken by one of her father's assaults, is so ugly that only plastic surgery could make her physically acceptable. She has left her husband, a tightly wired business colleague with whom no psychological dialogue was possible. She has begun a new relationship with a man who offers her much more intimacy and support. And she has taken an extremely challenging job with a consulting firm that places her on the cutting edge of many major political and economic issues.

Given her new responsibilities, Miranda is still not sleeping well, but she can sleep when she needs to because she uses her drugs in an intelligent way. She has a long-acting sedative for use three times a week, and a short-acting sedative for occasional use if she wakes in the night and cannot fall back asleep.

Miranda is as fully informed as I am about the chemicals she is using. And she knows how little we really know about how and why they work. But her life is on track. She doesn't smoke, her diet is balanced, she exercises vigorously, drinks moderately, and enjoys both her casual and intimate personal relationships with passionate enthusiasm.

Although she is a unique individual, Miranda's plight is legion. She epitomizes the conflicts confronting modern professional women. Furthermore, as she races to and fro her biological clock is ticking at the top of her brain stem. Sooner or later she will probably want children. To accommodate a full domestic agenda in her current life would require more change than all the pharmaceuticals in New Jersey could catalyze.

To get off the drugs completely, Miranda needs to learn to say no. She has difficulty in refusing excessive and inappropriate responsibility. She also needs to alter her schedule, sacrificing some of her activities. Miranda is not a short sleeper, but her schedule often forces her to become one. She must learn to let herself be the longer sleeper she really is. It takes some of us a long time to figure out where we belong on the key spectra that determine our optimal brain-mind states. Meanwhile we may need the help of a reluctant chemist.

Some readers might say, "So what if Miranda has to take these drugs the rest of her life. Diabetics take insulin every day." The difference is that Miranda's sleep loss is not life-threatening. Without drugs, diabetes is fatal. There is a cost for Miranda's regular use of drugs: dependency. She has a subtle addiction to the sedatives, and she will become habituated. She will need greater doses for the drugs to achieve the same effect. She will have a problem greater than insomnia. To be really cured, Miranda has to take full voluntary control of her life, and her brain-mind states, and get off the drugs.

NO DRUGS OR NEW DRUGS

Relief from symptoms is a strong motivator, strong enough at times that people like Miranda, who are informed, consciously choose to risk addiction and habituation. There is an even stronger force out there that motivates the uninformed to take drugs: profit. The pharmaceuticals business is one of the greatest moneymakers in history.

It is hard for people to resist advertising and to resist running to the drugstore for any number of remedies when they are in search of relief from a cold, or anxiety, or lack of sleep. It is hard, in part, because they are uninformed about what they are taking. The plethora of drugs on any given shelf of a drugstore to fight any one of the discomforts just mentioned is mind-boggling. Are they all necessary? Is one better than another? The answer to these questions is often no.

We do not need drugs to overcome many illnesses, especially mild mental ones such as sleep loss or anxiety. Even if we decide we do need a drug, we do not need a different drug for each illness. This myth is perpetuated by the FDA, which approves drugs in this way, and the pharmaceutical companies, which market drugs in this way.

Here's some proof. Go to the drugstore and pluck five medications for colds off the shelf, five for seasickness, and five for allergies. Read the labels. You'll find a long and differing list of sugars and binders and all sorts of nonsense. But the active ingredients are the same. They may have different trade names, but in fact they are all antihistamines. Some are phenothiazines. And remember what we used at The Psycho to calm Bertal? Chlorpromazine, which is not only an antihistamine but also a phenothiazine. The same group of compounds is used to relieve the dynamically different symptoms of cold, flu, hay fever, seasickness, and wild psychosis. One drug — and a generic one for that matter, which would be cheaper than a brand name — could replace an entire thirty-foot shelf of products at the pharmacy.

The same insidiousness goes on in psychiatry. The doctors on Park Avenue who counsel the high-strung elite who can't handle the "pressures" of high society fill their clients' medicine cabinets with Valium to control stress, Librium to control excessive drinking, and Dalmane to control sleeplessness. These are all benzodiazepines. They are the same base molecule, each with a little twist that makes a slight difference to the molecular action, and are prescribed in different dosages, colors, and flavors to make the whole act seem brilliantly selective.

Even if you accept this folly, the worst abuse is that doctors continue to prescribe, and patients continue to take, these drugs for years and years. Small wonder when you see the headlines in tabloids about a prominent public figure who has had a breakdown or is "suddenly" admitted to a rehab clinic.

Even if these individuals have serious problems, their doctors should prescribe drugs only as a temporary means to jolt them out of their state and should then turn to scientific humanism for the long-term cure. These individuals may need a drug for a few days or weeks to break their cycles, but then they must use volition to keep themselves healthy. Only volition can cure them. That's why groups like Alcoholics Anonymous work; there is a collection of people who mutually support each other. There is a collective will. Once the individuals in the group feel the power of their own volition, they can control their states, and the natural healing power of the mind and body will kick in.

Virtually all the drugs on today's market hurt some of the body's systems while helping others. Valium may reduce anxiety, but it also induces an obstinate case of drug dependency. Antihistamines may reduce sneezing, but they also make you sleepy, and they can put you into the kind of funk I entered when I took my roommate's cold pills before assisting in delivering babies.

Hope is near on the horizon. There is a growing list of impressive chemicals in trials that will not create the problem of addiction that stimulants and depressants present or the side effects that other drugs present. They accomplish this by working in a fundamentally different way.

A replacement for amphetamine may be at hand. Amphetamine is an amine molecule that looks enough like norepinephrine to fool the receptors on nerve endings. The receptors open the slips and lock in the amphetamine molecules. In depressed people, too few amines are reaching the receptor sites. The amphetamine stands in for norepinephrine, just as carbachol can stand in for acetylcholine. The problem is that amphetamine hits faster and harder and its action is more short-lived. Furthermore, its presence inhibits the production of amines even further, making the user more reliant on the drug in the future. Cocaine and "crack" are the current street names for this kind of drug. They are popular because they have the power to drive people sky high into energetic elation, and they are condemned because they can enslave their victims by their very power.

The better solution would be either to increase the number of amines produced or to extend their lifetimes while they are floating in the synapse, so their chances of finding a vacant receptor site are increased. Recall that acetylcholine is chewed up by cholinesterase when it is left in the synapse. The body regulates amines in the same way. A drug that could block the natural breakdown of amines, or could block the amines from returning to their home ports when they can't find a receptor, would improve the transmittance of signals by the amines, energizing the depressed patient.

The new drugs that act by blocking the return of the amines are called reuptake-blockers. They include Prozac, the upstart drug that has received so much recent attention due to its great success in relieving obsessive thinking and depression. For a reluctant chemist like myself, this is the sort of medicine I might be able to live with. Such new drugs potentiate the action of natural neurotransmitters instead of replacing them. Because they don't turn off the normal release, they do not initiate the addiction cycle.

Another class of the new drugs that achieves the same effect has the additional and surprising property of suppressing REM sleep without causing the usual buildup of tension, payback with interest, and breakthrough into waking that is seen in alcohol withdrawal. This remarkable feature was first noted during the treatment of narcolepsy with so-called monoamine oxidase inhibitors. These drugs increase the efficacy of norepinephrine and serotonin by blocking enzymatic breakdown. The net effect is the same: each aminergic molecule is more effective because it is longer-lived. And because the aminergic system is thus strengthened, the cholinergic system is more strongly inhibited. There is less REM suppression. For alcoholics in withdrawal, these drugs might reduce hallucinations and nightmares. For those who are depressed, these drugs would give them a lift while also eliminating dreaming.

The absence of dreaming, without a decrease in health, suggests that we may not need the dreams themselves to accomplish the physiological function that REM sleep provides — restoring the amines. Maybe dreams are really an epiphenomenon, a secondary and unnecessary outcome of an underlying process. Maybe they are not important psychological experiences. This conclusion is already suggested by the near total amnesia that we all normally have for our dreams.

But if the REM sleep is gone — along with the dreams — doesn't that mean that REM sleep is equally useless? At first glance it would seem so. Let us reflect on what the drug actually does. It increases the efficacy of norepinephrine and serotonin, which is the very purpose we ascribe to REM sleep — to give the aminergic system time off so it can restore its efficacy. If there is plenty of drug around — so much that the aminergic system is always efficacious — then REM sleep is not needed. Its function has been replaced by the drug.

Now that, to me, is an interesting idea. There are no dreams, because there is no REM sleep. There is no REM sleep because the drug keeps the aminergic system robust. The drug protects the aminergic system from the loss of efficacy that would normally occur during waking. The drug can take the functional place of both REM sleep and dreaming.

Those readers who have not already gone into rage at this barbarian assault on the sacred mystique of the dream may have a cool-headed follow-up question. What about the cholinergic system? If there is no REM sleep, isn't tension building in the cholinergic system? Doesn't the cholinergic system need the release it gets during REM sleep?

The answer to this very good question appears to be that many of the new antidepressant drugs are anti-cholinergic at the same time that they are pro-aminergic. They simultaneously quell the cholinergic system. Here is a case in which a so-called side effect of a drug may be a highly desirable main effect. Whether this suppression is dangerous in the long term remains to be seen. But if the drugs *replace* the need for the cholinergic system to release itself, instead of just suppressing the action, then there would be no negative effect.

The implications of these speculations are monumental. And perhaps a large part of the reason I am a reluctant chemist is that when I prescribe most drugs, I don't really know what I am doing. The more powerful and potentially efficacious the drug, the more I am intimidated, humbled, and cautious about prescribing it. I know too much not to realize how ignorant I am, and how much we still have to learn.

BERTAL'S WAY OUT

The fact is, our ignorance is dangerous to the patients we serve. We physicians, of course, are trying to do our best, but what we don't know *can* hurt our patients. I have carried a disturbing question around with me for thirty years, since I left The Psycho. Did we actually help Bertal? Or hurt him? Or both? And in what proportion were his benefit and his harm?

We already know how Bertal reached his state of crisis. Let me propose how we could have helped him, armed with what we've learned about the brain-mind paradigm in the decades since I last saw him.

First and foremost, it is clear to me that we made the mistake of putting the psychotherapeutic cart before the pharmacological horse. In Bertal's case, we should not have been such reluctant chemists. As soon as we saw that he was flagrantly psychotic, we should have treated him with a drug that could have immediately stabilized his state.

Chlorpromazine is such a drug. We just used too little, too late. If we had administered a rapidly increasing dose schedule from the first day he entered the ward, we could have repulsed his hallucinatory dive-bomber, melted his statuesque poses, and reined in his galloping sleep deprivation — which only made his psychosis worse. I daresay we could have spared my supervisor his black eye — but a part of me has to admit that he deserved it.

Practicing psychoanalysis on an untreated psychotic patient now seems to me to be at once the height of hubris and the nadir of naïveté. The insight Bertal gained at the hands of my free-associative psychotherapy seemed only to make him more anxious, not less. Inspired by Freud's theory that paranoid psychosis is caused by repressed homosexual impulses, we did our best to make Bertal aware that we thought he might have a closet gay spirit. The result was panic — and disaster — for Bertal and everyone else on the ward, as he reacted with rage and rampage to prove he was a real macho man.

Even is his psychotic confusion Bertal was trying his best to tell us to drop the interpretations. "I'm learning too much," he protested one day when he appeared on the ward with lips coated with hemorrhoidal cream. And then, prophetically, he added, "I only need one brain!" Meaning, I suppose, that he had enough to deal with without our adding to his anxious burden.

I now have no doubt that if we had immediately entered into a *chemical* dialogue with his *brain,* we could have obviated three months of painful, damaging, and unnecessary psychosis. Step one then would be to quickly reestablish state control by clamping down on Bertal's brain-mind. Call it a chemical straitjacket if you will, but do not withhold its merciful restraint from a raving catatonic. Resetting the level of Bertal's brain amines and acetylcholine with chlorpromazine could have stopped the psychotic music playing in Bertal's head as quickly as waking arrests our own dreams — and by perhaps the same mechanism: quenching the cholinergic fire.

Then, and only then, could he realistically and effectively turn his attention to the behavioral and psychological devices that we have learned so much about from Delia. Could he then tune in on his dreams? Why not? Even if we no longer care to interpret dreams in Freudian terms, we saw through Delia how directly informative they were of her continuing conflicts. As in Delia's case, Bertal might have been able to find his own reasons for wanting to distance himself from his overprotective and intrusive mother. He might then have been able to leave home, live alone, and seek a more mature love for himself.

Once his psychosis was under the control of medication, Bertal could have begun to find other means of reducing his anxiety. He could have learned the relaxation response and could have enhanced his sleep with exercise. He might even have learned the helpful trick that Harriet used to nip her delusions and hallucinations in the bud by envisioning the books in her library. Bertal could have increasingly brought his own brain-mind states, including his psychosis, under a voluntary control that was informed by the brain-mind paradigm. He would still perhaps not be fully free of his problem. But he would be well enough to function positively. And he would be well enough to seek the chemical, behavioral, and psychological help he needed to prevent a disastrous recurrence of his psychosis.

In this way we might have avoided the poignant dialogue that Bertal and I had the day before he was to be transferred to that 1960s graveyard for failed treatments, the Boston State Hospital. "I'm sorry I was ever cured," Bertal said sadly, understanding somehow that we had raised his awareness of his problem but could offer him no solution. "You should have left me in the dream world."